"Silence Your Fat Gene *offers practical approaches to weight loss and quieting the hidden triggers of fat gain. It's well known that proper supplementation, diet, exercise, and rest are the foundation of a sustained healthy lifestyle. Dr. Emran provides an easy-to-follow guide based on these truths. I highly recommend this book to anyone dedicated to conquering this epidemic."*

—*Solomon Gee, Director, Melaleuca.com*

Silence Your **Fat** Gene

Discover the Hidden Triggers That Cause Fat Gain and Shut Them Down for Good

Mohammad A. Emran, MD

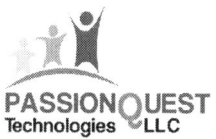

PASSION**QUEST**
Technologies LLC

Silence Your Fat Gene
*Discover the Hidden Triggers That Cause Fat Gain
and Shut Them Down for Good*

For information, or to order additional copies of this book, please contact:

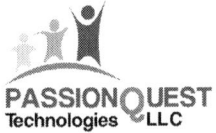

PASSIONQUEST
Technologies LLC

Phone: 707-688-2848
Fax: 707-402-6319
Email: info@earnprofitsfromyourpassion.com
5055 Business Center Dr., Suite 108, PMB 110, Fairfield, CA 94534

Interior book production by Cypress House
Cover design by 99designs/AleMiglio

Cover images:
DNA strand: Maxim Gaigul/Shutterstock.com
Silhouette: Nomad_Soul/Shutterstock.com

Publisher's Cataloging-in-Publication Data

Names: Emran, Mohammad A., author.

Title: Silence your fat gene : discover the hidden triggers that cause fat gain and shut them down for good / Mohammad A. Emran.

Description: First edition. | Fairfield, CA : PassionQuest Technologies LLC, [2017] | Includes bibliographical references.

Identifiers: ISBN: 9780991261147 | LCCN: 2017901091

Subjects: LCSH: Weight loss--Physiological aspects. | Weight loss--Handbooks, manuals, etc. | Weight gain--Physiological aspects. | Body weight--Regulation. | Fat cells--Physiological aspects. | Gene regulatory networks--Physiological aspects. | Biological control systems. | Metabolism- -Regulation. | Health. | Well-being. | BISAC: HEALTH & FITNESS / Diet & Nutrition / Weight loss.

Classification: LCC: RM222.2 .E577 2017 | DDC: 613.2/5--dc23

Printed in the USA
2 4 6 8 10 9 7 5 3 1
First edition

Dedication

To all those who have ever felt powerless against their weight, who have struggled with it over and over and wish to finally prevail. You are *not* just a product of your genes. You have the power within you to change their direction to a better and healthier one. Learn, apply, and repeat over and over. Silence Your Fat Gene and create the future you want. Bon voyage!

Permissions and Credits

Selected images used in this book are credited as follows:

Castle: "Huang Zusheng © 123rf.com"

Old Wooden Shack/Out-house: "Prill © Depositphotos.com"

Inflatable Bouncy Castle: "Nmorozova © Despositphotos.com"

Building Model on Blueprint Sheets:
"Maxim Kazmin © 123rf.com"

Radio dial: "ilze79 © 123rf.com"

Kitten: "Eleonora Vatel © 123rf.com"

Pile of fresh mango: "ConnyFuchs © Depositphotos.com"

Wild tomato bush: "Sheryl Caston © 123rf.com"

Protein gear: "ibreakstock © Depositphotos.com"

Protein lever: "ibreakstock © Depositphotos.com"

Clock gears: "thomaslenne © Depositphotos.com"

Cis bonds: "molekuul © 123rf.com"

Iguana lizard on branch: "fotoall © Depositphotos.com"

Cholesterol: "Anton Lebedev © 123rf.com"

Progesterone, Estradiol, Estrone, Theelol:
"Anton Lebedev © 123rf.com"

Androsterone, Dehydroepiandrosterone, Testosterone:
"Anton Lebedev © 123rf.com"

Normal and Rickets bones: "alila © 123rf.com"

Milo of Croton: "Patrick Guenette © 123rf.com"

Two Mice: Dolinoy, D.C., D. Huang, and R.L. Jirtle. 2007.
"Maternal nutrient supplementation counteracts bisphenol-A-induced DNA hypomethylation in early development,"
Proceedings of the National Academy of Sciences of the United States of America 104(32):13056–61.

Neuron: "designua © 123rf.com"

Toilet: "Elnuer_ © Depositphotos.com"

Lion standing: "Eric Isselee © 123rf.com"

Zebra: "Bernard Mackenzie © 123rf.com"

Contents

Acknowledgments

I thank my wife and children for their support throughout my mission to help people find a better way. Thanks to my team, Andrew and Stephanie, who keep me moving forward even when the shiny objects get distracting. Thanks Myron and Judy for being great friends and good students and for persevering—you have strength and conviction, now do what you know you have to do!

Introduction

Weight loss and weight gain are extremely emotional ideas. Despite their origins as personal challenges, they've destroyed lives, families, and even economies. Many people have been emotionally devastated or left with distorted views of their bodies. If these complex problems were simple, there would be one solution or leader in the weight-loss industry. Instead, there are thousands of diet programs, thousands of exercise programs, and thousands of weight-loss surgeons. No one has emerged as a real solution for everyone. While common features may help everyone lose weight, individual risk factors, history, psychology, and lifestyles create significant complexity and variation. One person can succeed with a particular product, system, or exercise and the next person may completely fail. The failure is not of the individual but the system, and the only time you fail is when you don't act. How can you achieve a healthy weight when the system doesn't work for everyone? The answer is to identify your risk factors for obesity and which ones have an active role in your life.

Have you dieted or tried to get fit by losing weight, or struggled with belly fat or cellulite? Have you had or thought about weight loss surgery? Have you seen the gimmicks to lose "twenty pounds in twenty days" and realized they were temporary fixes? Have you worked out for hours only to see little impact on how you look and lose body fat? Have you tried the shakes, bars, and prepackaged foods? You're not alone. Millions of people have yet to find a solution. The solution has not been easy to find because only one or two causes of weight gain were considered, or one or two foods that caused the problems. No one has probed the hidden factors that contribute to weight gain throughout the year.

Avoid the scams and "lose weight quick" schemes that don't work. You've seen weight-loss programs described as "scientifically proven" or labeled as "successful for thousands," but how do you know whom to believe? A simple method is to Google search the author, the name of the weight loss product, or the "before and after" photos they use. If your search results fail to find anything of substance, or worse, anything negative, simply walk away. If the review has a button to go to a product or program, it's not real. Walk away. These systems take a scientific discovery and turn it into hype: they use key words like "magic" and "quick" to attract people's attention. If eighty thousand people benefited from a program or diet the evidence trail would be easy to find, and someone with nothing to gain would talk about how great it was.

The natural process of weight gain starts fairly simply, and has been made more complex by the environmental factors you are exposed to. You can't point to someone and say, "You are overweight because you're lazy and eat too much." Doctors still do this, and so do friends and family. This is far from the truth for most people. Blame avoids the causes and ignores the risk you face when you gain weight and become unhealthy, and for your children as they develop in the same environment that breeds obesity and health deterioration. There are crucial concepts and information that can help stop this trend in you, your family, and your children. If you're ready to "try one more time" for a solution to obesity, keep reading.

Beginning in the Past

Let's go back in time to see how the problem of obesity developed and how it affects all of us. Ever since primitive times, people have searched for ways to make life on earth more comfortable, secure, and prosperous. We woke at sunrise and went to bed at sunset. We were in touch with our instincts about thirst, hunger, fatigue, and specific food cravings. We were constantly in motion when awake in our drive to catch, hunt, gather, harvest, plant, make, and create. There were few moments of idle time between these activities and this was filled with dancing or practicing to hunt and fight. The sunrise, sunset, seasons of harvest, and the seasonal migrations of animals determined the schedule we lived by. We traveled, worked, gathered, hunted, and harvested based on the seasonal clock. Over time, each person or family specialized in a few skills and we shared these skills to help everyone survive.

New ideas and inventions served to give us an advantage in survival and yet we remained linked to the world around us. We felt cold when it was cold, hot when it was hot. We sweated in the heat and shivered in the cold. When thirsty we drank, when hungry we ate. We had to make a physical effort to produce food by hunting or preserving it for later. We often ranged widely to do this. We sought shelter from the elements by covering in skins and hiding in caves. Later this progressed to clothing and homes, but we still relied on nature's abundance and were at the mercy of the elements. Eight hundred thousand years ago, we discovered the use of fire and this reduced energy needs in winter and helped unlock more energy from the food we ate. This also reduced some of the effort to feed and protect us.

As we specialized further, the population grew and survival was easier. More time was spent finding new ways to make life easier and more prosperous. Instead of mere survival, we tried to tame nature and our fears. We kept domesticated animals and no longer had to range. Ten thousand years ago the agricultural revolution happened, allowing us to extract more food from the area we lived in by cultivating the land. We learned to farm on a larger scale and no longer had to gather what nature provided. Instead, we guided and sometimes forced nature to produce what was demanded instead of what was needed. Eventually we made complex and efficient machines to do the labor that was once done by hand. These machines meant less physical work and more mental work. Better homes with heating meant easier winters. Air-conditioning meant easier summers. Grocery stores meant abundance. Less effort was required for daily survival and we no longer feared the elements or the predators now relegated to parks, zoos, and nature preserves.

During this process we extricated ourselves from the cycle as old as time. The changing of the seasons was the cycle to which life on earth had adapted to survive. By changing our position in nature, we were no longer beholden to the weather but set ourselves apart and established our new place in the world. We no longer ate what nature provided in the quantities necessary and at the times prescribed. We modified the animals and plants we ate to give them the characteristics we desired. We did this with crossbreeding and selection, and then by genetic modification. We never considered what we were giving up.

As a result, many first-world countries have seen the explosion of health problems such as obesity, diabetes, breast cancer, colon cancer, diverticulitis, asthma, eczema, attention deficient hyperactivity disorder (ADHD), autism, autoimmune disorders, and many more conditions. These are not seen in much of the third world, where people still depend on and participate in nature. In nations where the transition from third to first world has changed from the reliance and interaction with nature to the dominance of the natural world and exclusion from nature, you can see the same diseases appear. It is no wonder that obesity is increasing. All focus is on caloric, fat, and carbohydrate intake. But this is just scratching the surface of the problem of obesity. Many other hidden contributors exist and are relevant to solving the problem. Until these contributors are addressed, the obesity epidemic will continue.

The Problem Today

Obesity rates in the U.S. are predicted to grow to between forty-two percent and fifty-one percent of the population by 2030. This represents nearly $550 billion in additional healthcare expenditures over what we are already paying (Finkelstein, 2012). What are we paying now? Nearly $148 billion per year goes to direct obesity related cost, which represents at least 6.7 percent to 10 percent of each state's total medical expenditures. The taxpayer pays twenty to fifty percent of this cost (Trogdon, 2012). While the U.S. obesity rate is huge, the worldwide problem is colossal by any standards. The epidemic's rate of expansion has risen from 1.4 billion people in 2008 to over 2.1 billion in 2013. This contributes to international healthcare costs and results annually in millions of deaths. When you factor in that obesity is a symptom of poor nutrition and not just over-feeding, and look at all the obesity related conditions as well as those from the same poor diet—the costs are staggering.

As I share the unconsidered causes for obesity, scientific evidence is provided to support the argument that we have extracted ourselves from a critical place in nature and caused many of our own ailments by eliminating the normal environmental signals to gain and lose weight. There are many unsubstantiated claims about obesity and its cure. Someone says something and others repeat it without verification. In contrast, *Silence Your Fat Gene* has a reference section to let you verify the research and share with others who have similar questions and concerns. Remember, no matter the topic in science, there are always conflicting reports. You only get an accurate picture of what's going on by looking at the research as a whole and interpreting not just the experiments and observations but also how they were done. Keep in mind that what you see in the news is presented to stir up controversy, attract attention, or challenge accepted beliefs. Other stories are designed to drive product sales of fad drugs, supplements, and exotic extracts without adequate proof of efficacy and safety.

My first book, *Fast-Track Your Health: The Four Keys to Successful Weight Loss*, was a practical guide to organizing your weight loss effort. It had quite a bit of science to support the recommendations and the goal was to have a usable manual to help the person trying to achieve better health. Several readers told me they read it in a single day and used the material to achieve twenty, thirty, and fifty pounds of weight loss in a few short months without drastic changes in eating, exercise, or lifestyle. *Silence Your Fat Gene* provides similar practical pieces of advice for achieving your health but is designed to give you a fuller picture of how the natural interactions between you and your environment has been disrupted and how to restore your health through the balance nature intended. By addressing the hidden causes of obesity, you can lose the extra weight and start feeling healthier and more energetic than when you were twenty-five years old.

Silence Your Fat Gene gives suggestions about how to block the unconsidered causes of weight gain and restore your health. A list of weight-gain triggers is provided that allows you to determine your own risk profile. Not every trigger will be relevant to you. Some may not apply while other triggers are almost universal. As you read, you will find the ones that fit your situation and put you at risk for weight gain and poor health. I will show you how we have put ourselves into four seasons of fat gain while ignoring spring, the one season that provides a large part of the cure to what ails us. You can restart your path to health and wellness simply by harnessing the transformative attributes of spring. More precisely, I will share with you key signals that help you unlock the language of your cells and tell them to finally give up the fat for good.

Once you get your body into alignment with the natural processes that keep weight off it will be easier to pass the knowledge to your children. You'll live to see them and your grandchildren playing, graduating, and getting married. You will change your life, improve your relationships, and enjoy yourself rather than constantly obsessing, measuring, or worrying about what your next meal will do to your health.

Before going any further, I want to tell you exactly what you won't find in this book: New weight-loss pills, a magic supplement or new tropical jungle miracle berry; workouts; reviews on best shakes or meal replacements; recommendations to eat the same boring foods or packaged meals; dangerous-to-your-health quick fixes; and one-size-fits-all solutions. If you're excited by a practical way to identify the triggers for your personal weight gain, keep reading. If you're looking to achieve personalized, targeted weight loss, keep reading. If you are looking to not feel like you're starving, torturing your body, or doing things that are *unnatural* to lose weight, keep reading. The answers to your questions and the secrets to unlocking your fat gene are at your fingertips. This isn't an exhaustive report on the subject, but enough to give you the main ideas, provide resources and solutions, and get you moving toward your goal.

Again, there is no specific diet or exercise program here. *Silence Your Fat Gene* will help you identify specific targets for your personal weight loss and health improvement efforts, and the triggers for your weight gain to shut them down one by one. Certain chapters have sidebars in the margins that explain some of the more scientific terms being discussed. This allows you to skip the technical terms on a case-by-case basis. Most important is the concept that you have control over your destiny. If you're ready to take control and silence *your* fat gene, let's get started.

Building Your Castle

Your body under a microscope looks like it is constructed of tiny bricks: these are your cells and build a more complex structure. The structure is taken for granted and we don't often consider what goes in. Take a moment and think about how your body is built. The food you eat is the material that goes into its construction. We've looked at food incorrectly for three generations or more, and abandoned what our forefathers knew about the connection between nutrition and health. Currently, we think of food in terms of energy intake, but not what it provides in the way of nutrients. These nutrients are the materials used in maintaining your body.

The concept of your body as a temple is accurate, but I like to think of the body as a castle. How you think about your body has a huge impact on how you treat it. Your body is a castle and your defense against outside invaders. You can build it strong or weak. You can allow it to fall into disrepair or continually upgrade and improve it. To build a strong castle you need to be sure only the best materials are used. You have a picture in your mind of what a castle looks like, but take the time to imagine your own perfect body/castle.

Close your eyes and imagine standing in front of a full-length mirror. See yourself in perfect health, having lost the excess weight, and being in the shape you want to be in. You're smokin' hot in that new dress or suit! This is the image of your castle, the perfect, healthy you.

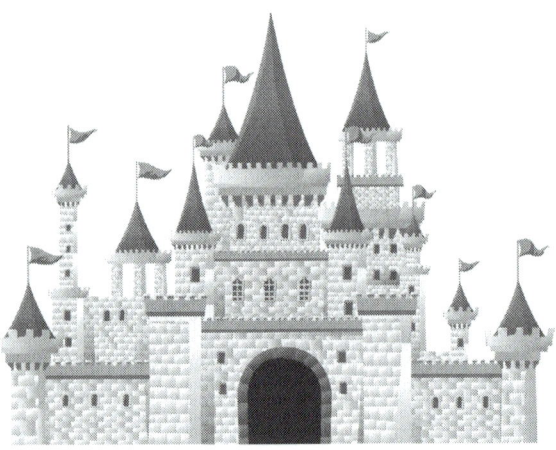

If your mind keeps resetting to the "now"—or an image less than perfect—you know there is a problem with your self-perception. Unless, of course, you are already in awesome shape and perfectly fit and healthy. If you can't get to the perfect image seek health coaching for assistance in making the breakthrough to see you're worth it (see Resources). To see your possibilities and create an image of your goal is crucial to your success. Now you have your castle blueprints!

With your castle blueprint complete, start thinking of the construction. What materials do you want? The best materials, and best help and advice will build the castle you want. Building the perfect castle isn't cheap, but it can be made affordable. Doing things right the first time keeps you from having to spend extra to fix problems later. Don't mistake convenient and cheap as a good alternative when on the go. Those materials are the equivalent of going to the junkyard, and make your castle weaker and less attractive. You don't want a castle that looks like a shack.

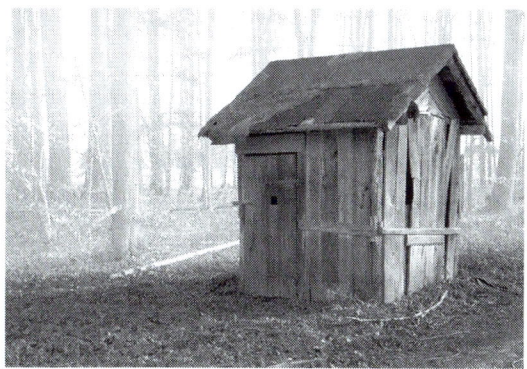

No matter how much paint and Spackle you put on the walls of a shack created from junk you will still not have a castle. Decorating and shaping can't turn the basic structure into what it's not. Every day, people choose bad advice and inferior materials to build their castles. Don't take advice from a clown on how to build your castle. Getting materials from the clown results in something that looks fun but has no real substance or strength.

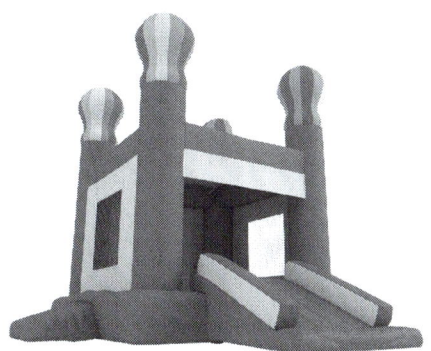

Choosing good materials on a regular basis, and from an early age, makes sure the construction is done right and it's solid and durable. Rebuilding or renovating a castle takes longer than building it right the first time. It's possible, but you have to stop damaging the castle and start replacing the bad with the good. If you've ever done home renovation, you know what a mess it can be. Home-makeover TV programs often show the hidden problems that add cost when you least expect it. Your weight loss transformation is much the same. You will find challenges and expenses along the way but the result when you step into your new body and health is well worth it.

Every day you make choices that have an impact on how your castle will look and stand up to weather and invaders. Sometimes the choices are based on cost alone and this is a great mistake. Always make sure the best materials go into your castle—bricks of gold and silver. You want strength and durability.

"But, Dr. Emran, making those high-quality decisions are expensive." *Yes, no, not necessarily* is my answer. On the surface, making decisions that are good for you may cost money in the short term, but like losing weight, you are looking at a long-term goal instead of what happens tomorrow or next week. Every decision to super-size a meal can cost as little as sixty-seven cents but costs over six dollars in expenditures for more food to feed bigger fat cells, more fuel to transport the extra weight of the meal when added to your body as fat, and healthcare spending. That's an almost one thousand percent return on investment in a very negative way. Turn this around and make healthy choices that save these costs and reap a one thousand percent profit instead.

Think about it this way: would you walk into a car dealership, buy a new car, pay full price, get only the tires and leave satisfied? I bet you would want the car you paid for. Yet, we accept this with health and nutrition. We pay full price for something that gets us nowhere near our goals. Maybe that's an extreme example, so let's tone it down a bit and see if it makes more sense: where do you live, somewhere hot or cold? Imagine what you need more in your car, the heater or air conditioner. Take the same car-buying scenario but you don't get air-conditioning or heat. If you had to pay a little bit more to get what you want and need, would you? I'm betting most of us want one or the other and would be willing to make a small additional payment to get what we really need.

Ultimately, you want a durable castle you can be proud of and keeps you safe and secure. Your choices will reflect in a positive way in your health and appearance. A good example of where cost is different from your initial perception is the meal replacement shakes and bars many people use in a weight loss program. At first glance, they seem expensive. When you consider what you are replacing the cost comes into perspective a little more. With the meal replacement shake, you might pay less than the coffee and muffin you would have picked up on the way to work—and that flavored coffee and muffin would have done harm to your health. Making healthy choices to build your castle stronger *is* affordable and will give you long-term savings as well.

I've had young, overweight athletes referred by doctors for health problems related to excess body fat and bad eating habits, only to have their coaches, trainers, or teammates convince them they shouldn't lose weight. They believe a heavier baseball player can hit harder and a heavier football player is better at defense. It's important to change the attitudes that put short-term, small gains before long-term major gains. An athlete wants more than a big castle, they also want it to look good, be strong, and last. A football player with a high body fat percentage who stops playing or is injured quickly gets deconditioned, gains additional weight, and starts having health problems. An increase in muscle and decrease in fat means better overall health and better performance. Football players aren't the only ones to suffer this pressure. Female softball players face the same kind of pressure to stay "bulked up." Unfortunately, it's not always muscle they are carrying.

Part of a castle's defense is the drawbridge and moat. In your body, you have to use defenses too. "Choice" and "judgment" are your drawbridge and moat. They determine what you eat, drink, and are exposed to. When you choose to only let in the good you are less likely to have problems in your castle and more likely to keep it safe and secure. Exercise fits into this analogy. Exercise is the cleaning, painting, maintenance, and decorating in the castle. Having a strong castle is great but you also want it to look good.

Remember though, no matter how much paint and cleaning, you can't turn a shack into a castle. The materials aren't there. This is why you need nutrition *and* exercise. To make a drastic renovation for your castle you have to take drastic action and add great materials. Your body is the same. With new stones, mortar, and hard work your castle can be transformed into what you want. The process requires planning, looking for the right materials, and doing things in the right order. Weight loss requires a similar process. You start with planning and learning what contributed to your weight gain. In *Fast-Track Your Health*, I talked about organizing the information and turning it into a plan of action with accountability. Imagine paying a contractor to renovate your castle without giving them a deadline. If they're paid by the hour rather than the result, guess how long it will take.

The castle analogy really becomes helpful when you ask about its maintenance. The cleaning, heating, and cooling take an incredible amount of time and resources. A better body requires similar attention in time, focus on excellent nutrition, and systematic progress toward the goal. Imagine cleaning out an old castle overgrown with weeds and full of rats and dust. Sound like fun? How long would it take to restore it to its former glory? Can you get it back to where it was? Yes, but with a tremendous amount of work, time, and cost. You have to fix the holes in the walls before you start painting and hanging tapestries. Yet, every day, people run to the gym without first paying attention to their nutrition.

Okay, did I just call your body a weed and rat-infested, broke-down castle? That's taking it a bit far, I know, but how many days have you woken up feeling like your head was full of cobwebs? How many people do you know who didn't maintain their castle only to have a wall suddenly collapse—like a heart attack or stroke? Have you or anyone you know tried to start the renovation process only to get hung up on details? We have to get past this. I did, my patients do, and you can too! Start maintaining your castle and start renovating it to be what you want!

When building your castle, always keep in mind the choice of what materials to use and the effort you put into maintenance is your responsibility. Be conscious of what decisions you make. Do you *really* want to achieve weight loss? If so, nothing will stand in your way. Never accept your contractor saying, "Sorry I can't get this exact hinge for your door so I can't renovate the rest of the castle," or let a missing window or stone stop progress. You and the contractor will find a way to make it work. Find other methods and materials, or more help to solve the problem. Your body and health deserve no less. If you aren't happy with the results you're getting, find a new contractor.

You can choose between the spooky, wicked witch castle and the pretty, princess castle. This depends on the materials you choose. Bargain basement and the best materials have very different results. A castle given a lot of care and attention will attract a prince, princess, or inspire someone in your life to treat you like one. On the other hand, the wicked witch castle might attract trolls and bloodsuckers. I know, silly analogy, but it *will* stick with you! Build a strong castle and the people around you with weak castles will change theirs. Most neighbors unconsciously compete, so compete in something positive.

I want to carry this analogy a little further because it will give you insight on how you can start making weight loss easier and your health better. Old-time castles weren't just a big house for the king, instead they represented a safe place for all the subjects. There was often a wall around a small village. Our body is like this with all our cells being the villagers that take refuge in this castle keep. This will become more important for our discussion later, but for now just think about these villagers in your castle. Each has a job and they share a common language. Now imagine for a minute being able to speak that language. Imagine being able to tell them to lose fat or build muscle on command. What if we've been speaking that language all along, but unknowingly telling our cells to gain weight instead? That is where all the fat triggers I will share later come in.

3

Reasons for Weight Gain and the Fat Gene

How does weight gain happen? Readers of my first book, *Fast-Track Your Health*, might recognize some of the following information. The research for that book led me to make a more thorough study of the causes of weight gain. I knew some of my patients failed to lose weight after reducing their calorie intake to a healthy level. They ate much less and yet continued to gain weight, while others had no problem losing extra pounds. Most eliminated many of the junk foods and yet the weight kept coming. Some lost weight only to regain it later. I decided to write this book to explain why this happens, how we've thought about weight loss in the wrong context, and how this has prolonged the obesity epidemic. More importantly, by looking at the reasons for weight gain you can identify new ways to combat the triggers at work in your body. I will show you many of the causes of weight gain and what you can do to fix them.

The balance of weight gain and weight loss has three components:

1. Dietary intake
2. Metabolism
3. Activity

Normally, all three are in balance. By changing or ignoring one factor the balance is disrupted, leading to weight gain. Dietary intake and activity are accepted as the factors that can be changed, but metabolism can also be changed.

Dietary intake is everything you eat or drink, and the source of calories that go into your body. Healthy intake must be balanced with the energy expenditures. Dietary intake must contain the appropriate nutrients for your body to function properly. Proteins, carbohydrates, and fats are essential components of the diet and play significant roles in health. Proper body functioning and use of energy requires vitamins, minerals, and water. If the intake is not adequate or excessive, this must be balanced by the other two factors. If your intake is too much or has too many unhealthy foods, you tip the balance toward weight gain. Unhealthy foods are those that have many calories but little nutrition. Even healthy foods can become unhealthy when they are repeated too much in your diet. This happens when they limit the opportunity for other nutrients. When your stomach is full of apples, you can't eat strawberries. When your stomach is full of lettuce, you can't eat meat.

According to the Centers for Disease Control the calories in the average American diet have increased as much as twenty percent in the last thirty to forty years, although the current awareness and push for health has started reversing this trend a bit (Ford and Dietz, 2013). The increase was most pronounced in women with over twenty percent and less for men at under ten percent. Most of these extra calories come from snacking on processed, carbohydrate-rich foods. That means taking in as much as three hundred to four hundred extra calories per day. This can add up to an extra pound of weight gain every ten days!

Calories are thought of as energy, like gas for a car, but this idea is flawed. If you keep the number of calories you need, regardless of where they came from, you get extremely different results. For instance, two thousand calories from spinach, broccoli, and kale isn't the same as two thousand calories from a hamburger and French fries. Two thousand calories of meat versus two thousand calories of sugar or two thousand calories of oil are very different. Calorie density, nutrient content, water content, fiber content, and the vitamins and minerals are very different. Each has an impact on your body functions and metabolism.

Cooked or raw food also determines the calories available. Cooked meats and vegetables release more energy than raw foods (and in some cases more nutrition), with the difference being ten to twenty-five percent (Carmody et al., 2011; Wrangham et al., 1999). Salad has fewer available calories than the same vegetables cooked. Sushi is harder to digest and has fewer calories than cooked fish. Your energy intake is widely affected by cooking, and in turn affects your metabolism.

Metabolism is the rate at which your body uses energy from your diet or the stored energy from your body to carry out normal body functions. This includes growth, healing, breathing, heartbeat, intestinal function, brain function, and more. While many people believe that metabolism is a fixed number, metabolism can be changed depending on your health, activity, and weight. This factor commonly sabotages many people's efforts at weight loss. By ignoring the effects of restrictive dieting and the need for proper nutrition to maintain metabolism, weight loss efforts can be doomed from the outset. Your metabolism is continuous. This is the greatest energy you use all day long. Having a slow or broken metabolism makes any efforts at weight loss difficult or impossible.

The final component in the balance of weight gain and weight loss is the level of activity. This comprises what you do on a daily basis as well as any exercise you add to your routine. The greater your activity, the more energy is expended. By increasing activity, you tip the balance toward energy loss and make weight loss easier. Even modest increases in activity can have dramatic results for your health. Diet, metabolism, and activity are all interlinked. For example: you can boost your metabolism by improving your diet and building muscle with exercise to improve your conditioning.

Energy Down the Drain

Metabolism determines how fast your body uses the calories you eat. To help you visualize the balance between energy intake, metabolism, and exercise, consider it like an old-fashioned bathtub with water as the food or calories you fill your body with. The open faucet is your energy intake. Like eating, the water flow fills the tub (potential weight gain). The drain represents your metabolism, and how quickly you empty the water from the tub. Water draining from the tub is just like your metabolism using calories for everything you do including your heartbeat, breathing, and brain function.

The drain isn't the only way to get water out of the tub. Those with children know how easy it is to splash water out of the tub. This splashing and movement is the exercise that helps decrease the amount of water in the tub and the amount of calories remaining in your body. The drain can become clogged and slow down, just like certain food choices and eating habits can do to your metabolism. Similar to the belief you cannot alter your metabolism, the drain may appear to have a fixed size—but this isn't true. You can clean out the drain, remove the plug, or even make it bigger. For your metabolism, this is done through consistent, healthy food choices and regular exercise.

Many people gain weight or struggle to take off the excess they have even while eating foods considered healthy. That means the three factors can't be all there is to the story. There has to be a deeper cause of why we gain weight and keep it on. We look to other countries or regions that have longer life spans and try to mimic their diet by picking the foods they eat and say these must be healthy. How many people have switched to olive oil and sushi? The answer is not just in the foods, even though some have healthy properties. The real answer is hidden in the combinations of foods in relation to the timing of their seasonal appearance in nature and many more hidden messages from the environment.

Environment contributes a lot to weight gain as does a big psychological component passed along from previous generations. Hardships suffered during times of famine or cold have imprinted the idea of having "extra weight" for survival. This idea of having a little extra weight was true before modern food supplies, antibiotics to treat illness, insulated homes, and warm clothing. Those who carried the most excess weight were the most successful hunters or farmers and later the wealthy. Gaining weight showed your health and later your wealth. But this led to the health problems we see today. This generational memory has stayed long after the need for excess weight and contributed to many people's weight gain. Fortunately, that memory is slowly being lost as awareness of the obesity problem grows.

The low fat diet promoted from the 1980s to 2000s has proven to be a colossal failure. Every diet, pill, or exercise fad is short-lived. They provide temporary benefits but great risks. Much science is behind why most interventions don't work. Learn what doesn't work for your weight loss and why, and avoid them in future efforts. The science is available—you just have to apply it on a regular basis. By looking at other contributions to weight gain and weight loss you can find the pieces that have an impact on your life and modify them to get the best results. For example, it's counterproductive to eat a low carbohydrate diet when you've already tried it without any benefit. The answer is different for everyone, and lies in the impact of many contributing triggers. By organizing a personal health improvement plan (see Resources), you can fight against their effects.

The problem you must overcome is admitting you don't know the cause or solution to your weight gain. You've been told, trained, and convinced of certain facts that are inaccurate and may cause more weight gain. It's much more complicated than just the energy in and out of the bathtub above. The picture you have of how your weight gain has happened and how your weight loss will become a reality is not accurate! Your understanding is based on incomplete information that you have been fed by a weight loss industry mostly interested in profits.

It's okay—everyone suffers from this problem of understanding in one area or another in trying to comprehend the complex world. Using incomplete information, we try to piece together a mental model of how things work, but the model isn't always accurate. Think about this for a second, try this exercise: Draw a picture of a bicycle. Take a minute and do this exercise. Did you do it? Does it look like it would work? Did you know that more than seventy percent of people can't complete the drawing even though they may own or ride a bicycle? Once you open your mind to the possibility that the model in your head is incomplete and there are new ways to make weight loss faster, easier, and more permanent the process becomes more fun and the goals easier to achieve.

Gaining Weight by the Season

Everyone is trying to find "one" solution to the obesity epidemic. They look for the "fat gene" that would solve the entire problem. Some scientists have made their life's work out of looking for this part of our genetic code that predicts who will be fat, why, and how to reverse obesity. The reality is we *all* have the fat gene. It is built into every animal as part of the mechanism to survive hardship. It has allowed us to survive famine, drought, and the normal seasonal changes of fall to winter and back to spring.

One of my patients was having a real struggle to lose weight. She ate better, exercised regularly, and yet still failed to lose weight. She told me she felt like her fat gene was turned on and asked if there was some way to turn it off. When I heard this, I started thinking, "If we all have the fat gene and it's a normal survival mechanism, what would turn it on?" What has an impact on the expression of this gene? Is there something we are exposed to that turns it on? How do we shut it off? I started looking at what can turn on a particular gene and whether modifying those factors could shut it off. I also wanted to know why the gene was so susceptible to being turned on.

To answer those questions, I looked to what turns on the fat gene in nature. Key triggers are hardwired into every animal. At the end of summer and the start of fall, animals see a change in the foods available to them. The nutrients in plants shift with the changing seasons. No longer are fresh greens, fruits, vegetables, and meat as readily available. Instead, many animals change toward fat-gaining diets that have less nutrition and more calories. The scarcity in nature starts the normal process of weight gain by shifting the diet and affects the metabolism. Fat gain helps animals survive the long winter ahead during potential hibernation. By limiting food sources to high-calorie, low-nutrient food sources, or by limiting total calories, we replicate the conditions necessary to initiate the same system of fall weight gain.

Understanding the impact of how you eat, your size, and physical activity on your metabolism gives you an additional tool to achieve weight loss. During weight loss, it is important not to limit dietary intake too much. Very restrictive diets ultimately lead to the body perceiving scarcity. This will slow your metabolism and make further weight loss very difficult or impossible. It may lead to more weight gain with continued restriction or even after the restriction is removed. This begins to touch on the mystery quality about food. Why does our modern diet lead to such profound weight gain? Why don't we achieve the anticipated results after adding healthy foods and eliminating the unhealthy? The reason for weight gain is not as obvious as once thought.

Rural societies where people are more tied to the seasons, nature, agriculture, and the sun have a cycle of weight gain and loss similar to other animals. The natural triggers to encourage weight gain act on rural people and they lose weight due to hard work and exposure to elements just like their animal counterparts. This seasonal weight variation can be greater than sixteen pounds in some populations (Lloyd, 2013; Sabbağ, 2012; Panter-Brick, 1995). Pat yourself on the back if you hold your weight steady and avoid that potential gain. Now, imagine if the modern diet, modern exercise, and modern exposures to environmental triggers cause the same weight gain throughout the entire year. Imagine that you never have the triggers for fat loss that balances this out. You can see this scenario leads to rapid weight gain and a challenge in maintaining a healthy weight.

Sugar Ain't So Sweet

One trigger for weight gain is how modernization has changed food from what used to be seen in rural society. Much of the modern diet has a higher composition of processed meats, refined fats, and—most important—refined starches and sugars. Fewer whole foods are eaten in exchange for components reassembled for better shelf life, better taste, easier manufacturing, and easier shipping. Processing also strips nutrition from food. A good example of this is table sugar or sucrose. This is one of the simplest substances we eat on a regular basis. The quantity of sugar consumption has increased dramatically over the past two centuries from less than ten pounds per year per person up to a whopping one hundred pounds per year per person, or more.

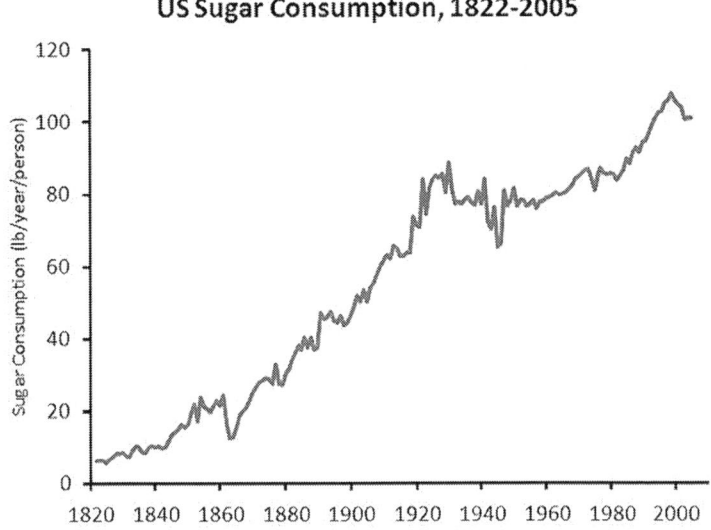

US Sugar Consumption, 1822-2005

Modern sugar goes through carbon filtration as well as ion exchanges to eliminate any particles and the natural brown color (see Resources). The resulting product is pure sucrose without the nutrients from the plant. We've stripped away the chewing and digesting required with sugar cane and beets. The sweet liquid extract that remains is then further purified to make sugar.

One important nutrient from sugar cane and beets is chromium. Chromium is a mineral that helps the body regulate sugar levels. Nature provides sugar along with this to help in regulating. Often in nature, the poison and the cure are in close proximity. Once the chromium is taken out, you are left with only the poison minus its cure. This lack of a key nutrient throws off the body's ability to control sugar levels or detect season and determine if weight gain should happen or the sugar be burned off for energy. This is only one example of a nutrient absence. In general, the lack of nutrients with excessive calories is what I refer to as the "fall diet."

Other things signal animals to gain weight besides nutrients. During the seasonal changes that happen through the year, animals adapt to different conditions. Seasonal changes also have a tremendous impact on how animals use energy. When the temperature drops in fall, winter is coming soon. Fewer hours of daylight and a change in temperature as fall progresses contribute to how much an animal eats and how it stores fat.

Today, we are rarely exposed to nature when it comes to temperature and lighting. We put ourselves in air-conditioned, low artificial light settings mimicking fall through every season. To this we add the fall diet, creating the worst possible combination of factors for maintaining healthy weight. We ready our bodies for hibernation. It's not surprising to start gaining weight similar to other animals preparing for winter. The problem is winter never arrives for us as it does for animals. We are never exposed to extreme cold or get to hibernate, and so the weight gain cycle never stops. We never have to keep warm with only our activity or body fat so the weight never leaves. We keep ourselves in a perpetual fall preparing for a winter that never completely arrives and a spring that is just a memory. Add this to chronic fatigue, chronic stress, lack of activity, and nutritional deficiencies and you have a witches' brew for weight gain.

Not only do the signals change how your fat genes are expressed but (and here is the scary part) they also have an impact on how your children's genes are expressed as well. We primed them to have characteristics like us. So, if you participate in behavior that is unhealthy, or eat a diet that causes excess weight gain, your children learn the same behavior and bad choices. You also modify your genes and contribute the same risk to your unborn children because they get the same modified genes. This makes a lot of sense from a survival standpoint. You can stop this process and turn off the fat gene. The answer to regaining your health and stopping the cycle of passing obesity to your children is spring. Spring is the cure. Since we don't hibernate, the only time to lose fat outside of winter is spring and early summer. Keeping your metabolism in spring and early summer counteracts the fall weight gain. The following chapters explore these concepts in more detail and look at the compelling evidence that supports this theory. Each aspect of the manmade fall will be considered, along with solutions that you can easily apply to change your life and health.

The Fat Gene

Some of the genes related to obesity (O'Rahilly, 2006) are also associated with syndromes, diseases, and conditions that cause other problems as well. There are eleven single mutations, fifty positions in the human genome for syndromes associated with obesity, and two hundred and fifty-three known genetic variations associated with obesity. Despite these spots on our deoxyribonucleic acid (DNA) and all of the known syndromes, this still accounts for only about one to five percent of all obesity (Li, 2010). That leaves ninety-five to ninety-nine percent unexplained by simple genetics! Something more must be going on.

Fat genes include those for fat storage, activity, internal clock, and appetite. We have yet to discover other categories, but these we know so far. I once heard a colleague deliver a beautiful presentation on the genetics of obesity. People sat entranced, hearing about the various regions of our genetic code that have an impact on weight. They were fascinated that so many things could go wrong and show up as obesity. It was interesting and intriguing. The problem was most people concluded they were overweight because of an undiscovered gene that doomed them to an eternity of spare tires and struggles with sugar cravings.

This outlook is fatalistic. "There is nothing I can do to change my genes, so I should do nothing." This is defeating yourself before you even try. It makes as much sense as a chicken breaking her own eggs because the fox got into the henhouse (okay, that was a Texas farm analogy, but you get the picture). It doesn't make sense to drive toward a cliff faster because there *might* be a cliff in your future. Don't give up before you start because someone tells you that the risk of obesity can't be changed. Understanding the genes and what they mean toward your weight loss is important only to a certain extent.

Many people interpret the studies showing maternal and paternal obesity contribute forty to seventy percent to the genetic risk of their child being obese as meaning the child is doomed to obesity. They read about childhood obesity determining what happens in adulthood and see this as proof that your parents give you fat genes and you can't change them once we get them. Heredity clearly has a role, but what is that role? Childhood obesity is rampant, but how much is actually due to your genes? Do we carry the risk of obesity from childhood into adulthood?

The normal time for the lowest fat-content in the body is five to six years of age. This drop is followed by an increase called the adiposity rebound. If this comes earlier, you have a much higher risk of obesity. If you're overweight by this time you are more likely to be overweight as an adult (Cunningham, 2014). While your risk is higher, the answer is more than having or lacking the fat gene. It is not fate. These are just numbers telling you what your risk may be. It is like saying your risk for dying in a car accident is higher if you're not wearing your seatbelt. The majority of people decide to wear the seatbelt to reduce the risk. This analogy carries into weight loss, weight gain, and your health. Everyone has the fat gene, but what separates those who gain weight from those who don't? The answer is even your genes can be changed or, more accurately, modified to turn on or off. With this knowledge, put on your seatbelt and reduce your risk of the car wreck of weight gain and health problems.

You can change your "fat fate" and what your genes predict you will do. Your DNA is just a blueprint and not "you." You are what you make of yourself from the materials in your environment. Picking your materials wisely and avoiding the things that trigger the fat genes is how to keep moving in the right direction. Finding out what things drive your weight gain or your health risks can help you address your personal challenges. Each of you has your own specific risk factors as well as those that are common to everyone. As you read this book, take note of the triggers that have a role in your life and put this information into a personal plan for improving your health. This will be finding the words in your body's language that will help you to tell it to stop gaining and start losing fat. Think of this book as a driver's education class for your body. You might have made a few mistakes like when you were learning to drive, but you will learn methods, learn to read the road signs, and get the tools to be a better driver to get to your destination quickly and, most important, safely.

4

Modifying Your Fat Gene

One presentation I gave about our ability to change our genes made several people perk up in the audience. They heard something they had never heard before. Some were very interested and others waited for the chance to tell me I was completely wrong. I posted an article online about changing your genes and was surprised at how many people sent angry comments. I received similar comments after I had a TV interview about fat fate and a person's risk of being overweight being set by the time they were five years old (Cunningham, 2014). I explained that the risk was only a number and you could change your risk by your behavior and choices. People didn't listen to that part of the interview and only heard about risk being set by the age of five. They criticized this as providing people with an excuse not to be healthy and any doctor who agreed with me was ignorant and shouldn't be allowed to practice medicine. We shouldn't use science as a replacement for personal responsibility nor should we ignore the valuable information science provides.

Unfortunately, that selective hearing and immediate jump to conclusions has led many people to wrong beliefs about weight loss, and worse, made them say things that led others astray. I'm a big proponent of scientific research and discovery. I rarely give advice or change my practice without having the science behind what I do. I know, however, that the findings of a study do not necessarily mean what people think they mean. In fact, they often don't support the author's conclusions, which are often jumps in logic that may not be true. The findings are often very clear but what they mean is usually less so. Even when authors of a study get unexpected results, they often try to explain this away or fit it into their belief system. Ignoring data and jumping to conclusions without an understanding of the whole picture is never a good idea. For an example of how wrong conclusions can cause devastating problems we only have to look to the late 1960s when a Senate committee was convened to look at the cause of increased heart disease in the U.S.

In 1968, the United States Senate Select Committee on Nutrition and Human Needs, also known as the McGovern Committee, was organized to research and improve malnutrition in children. The Committee quickly changed its focus due to concerns about the role of fat and cholesterol on American health. In reality, the focus changed because senators were concerned about their colleagues dropping dead of heart attacks and they wanted recommendations to reduce their risk. Many leading scientists (Oppenheimer and Benrubi, 2014) testified in their areas of expertise and came to conclusions that were incorrect. The question asked by the Committee was, "What causes heart attacks?" and the response was "Blockage of the coronary vessels." This was followed by "What blocks those vessels?" and the response was "plaques." The natural follow-up was, "What are the plaques made of?" and the answer was "cholesterol." "Where does cholesterol come from?" Saturated animal fat. The conclusion was saturated animal fat has cholesterol, cholesterol is in plaques, plaques cause coronary occlusion, coronary occlusion causes heart attacks, so animal fat and cholesterol are bad and we should eat a diet low in saturated fat and cholesterol. True, true, true, true, and unrelated.

What followed was a series of bad recommendations leading to an increase in heart disease, diabetes, and obesity. They had many facts that were true but their conclusion was wrong and unrelated. The same has happened with thinking about genes and genetics. Many wrong conclusions have entered into the collective psyche, which has distorted how we have looked at disease and heredity over the last fifty years. Look at what happened to the obesity risk after the recommendations, yet no one who made the recommendations backed off or reconsidered until just recently. Now, I've simplified this story a little but you get the general idea.

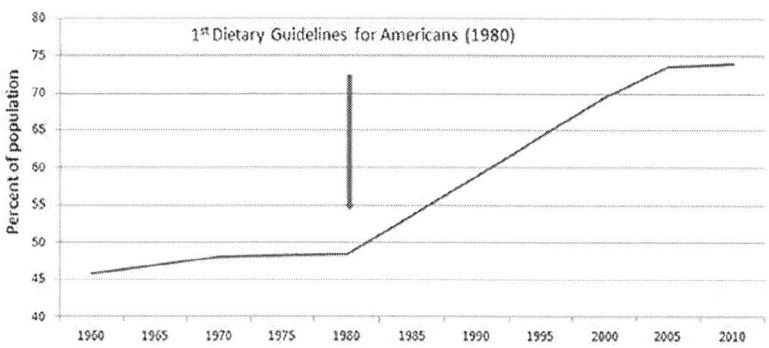

Age-Adjusted Percent of Population with a BMI ≥ 25 kg/m2
NHES and NHANES data (1960 – 2008)

Just after the recommendations we saw the risk of being overweight rise dramatically. Instead of less than fifty percent of Americans being overweight, suddenly the rate of being overweight rose consistently until exceeding seventy percent! Did we suddenly gain new obesity genes in America? Did mutation from nuclear testing put us at risk of gaining weight? No, obviously neither was true. New genes don't just show up in humans and cells have a powerful ability to fix mutations or errors in the DNA code. If they can't fix the damage they also have a failsafe called apoptosis that causes cells to commit suicide when their DNA is irreversibly damaged. If it is not new genes or mutations causing the rise in obesity, then what is it?

It's true that we get our genes from our parents, one set from Mom and one from Dad. The actual genes don't change. On the surface, this implies that no one has an impact on who she or he will become, what diseases they will have, or how long they will live. The reality is, it's not that simple. There's more to heredity and inheritance of characteristics than meets the eye. The specific question of cholesterol and fat is addressed later, but for now let's look at the other factors in genetics that are on everybody's mind.

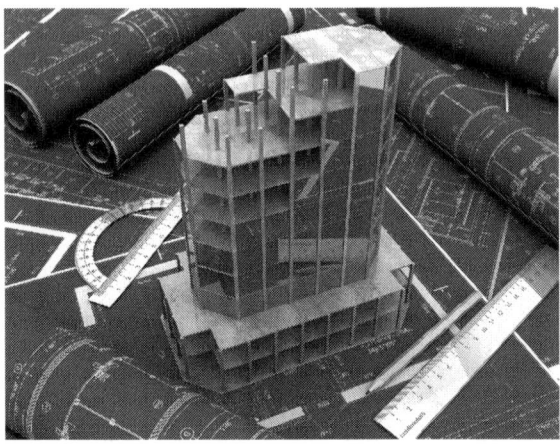

Previously, we considered genes as being either present or absent to determine our characteristics. We thought of the genetic code as a blueprint for who we would become, and our genes were a guideline that determined health, characteristics, and behavior. The problem with this concept is that genes don't turn themselves on or off and are not active all the time. Every cell doesn't need every gene active at the same time. Some genes have specific functions or deal with specific threats and challenges. For instance, it doesn't make sense for cells to be producing insulin when no sugar is present. Further, it makes no sense for insulin production in the cells in our bones. Instead, cells have a mechanism to turn on the specific parts of our DNA when they are needed.

A Roomful of Cats

The concept of a rigid blueprint is not an accurate description of how DNA works. When you are young and haven't been exposed to much in life, your genes determine who you are at that time. As you age, this changes. Your environment plays a bigger role. In fact, genes determine only one third of your characteristics. That leaves two thirds based on your experiences, actions, and exposures to the environment in which you live. Instead of a blueprint, your genetic code is more like an old-fashioned radio with two dials—a tuner and a volume. Each station on the tuner dial is one of your genes. Certain environmental stimuli can tune to a particular station and turn the volume up or down. A rigid blueprint won't let you react to changes in the environment. By having a system that is adjustable, you can better survive hardship and variable conditions. Your genes are turned on and off when and where they are needed.

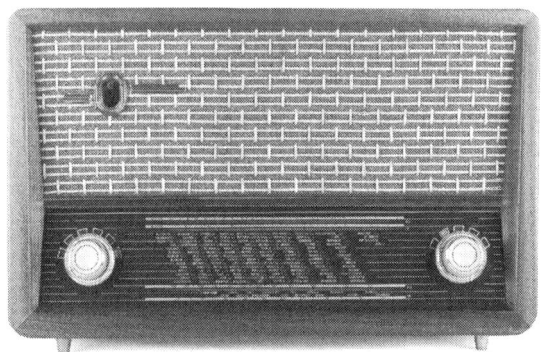

The problem with your radio is that it is sitting in a room full of cats. Now, wait, I know that sounds weird, but stay with me. Anyone who owns a cat knows they bump into things on the shelves all the time. A radio sitting on the shelf in a room full of cats has the tuner and volume being bumped at random. Certain genes are picked outside of your control when the tuner is bumped and the volume is turned up or down activating or inactivating that gene. The "cats" are the things you are exposed to in your environment. The man in front of you at the stoplight with exhaust pouring from his car into yours is a CAT. The coworker who brings doughnuts to work is a CAT. The cold you caught from your child going to school is a CAT. Many things in your environment have an impact and seem outside of your control.

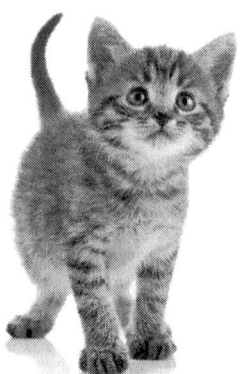

Everything you eat, drink, and breathe, and have contact with, are the cats tuning your radio dial seemingly at random. They seem innocent enough but behind that nonthreatening face are teeth and claws that can scratch the eyes out of your health. Even the light you are exposed to, radiation in the environment, sound, and nutrition can affect how your genes will be activated or inactivated. Ever wonder why members of the same family may have slightly different shades of the same eye or hair color? It's not just the combination of genes, but also how the environment has acted on them—or, which cats have bumped their radio.

As scientists learn more about how genes are expressed, they see many ways in which genes are modified by the environment you live in, causing them to be expressed differently. An entire area of science, epigenetics, looks at how DNA can be modified, activated, or turned off by environmental stimuli. This means there's good news about nature, healthy eating, and avoidance of unhealthy foods. The bad news is it not only affects how you feel and look in the short term but can have a great impact on which gene will be active. *What!? Yes, that's right.* What you eat or are exposed to in the world around you can affect how your genes are expressed, and even more frightening, which genes are expressed.

A number of years back, scientists got chickens to grow tails and teeth like dinosaurs. The genes were always there, they just weren't expressed until the scientists exposed the embryos to the right mixture of substances. With the right stimuli, an organism can dramatically change from what it was meant to be into something else. Given the right push you can change yourself. Which direction the push happens is important. Exposures and choices give the push, and while some may be out of our control, most are within our grasp to change. Substances absorbed by our cells will attach to our DNA to make genes more or less active. Sometimes this can be helpful and lead to an advantage to survive. The dark side is the risk that you get a bad feature like high blood pressure or cancer when exposed to the wrong things.

The obesity epidemic begins to make sense in the scope and rapidity with which it appeared. Back in the 1950s and 1960s there were few, if any, families who could claim that the entire family was obese. Today it is common to hear people say, "I come from a fat family" as an explanation for their weight gain. Some say, "I have the fat gene." Looking at their families in old pictures it is rare to see obesity before the 1980s. Even then, a rare family member was overweight and never to the present extent. Excess weight used to be a sign of wealth and success and only the elite suffered the diseases of obesity. Kings, senators, and wealthy businessmen gained the weight as a symbol of their success and excesses. It was rare for the average person, let alone a laborer, to be overweight. How has this changed? All of the previously mentioned stimuli play a role, but one more item remains. Genetics does affect weight but not how most people think.

How Genes React to Environment

Fat gene scientists and doctors have looked for that one gene that's the cause of weight gain. You know, the one that is supposed to be the target for a magic pill. Ironically, everyone has this gene or a combination of genes that allow us to gain weight. Your body has the built-in ability to survive hardship, bad weather, and famine, and stay alive with little food. We evolved to live in extreme conditions and have done so. It makes sense that the gene can be turned on when needed and off when it isn't necessary. Unfortunately, modern diet, activity, chemistry, and behavior have created multiple opportunities for the gene to act in inappropriate situations. Exposure to certain substances in the environment can contribute to obesity. This is not just by too many calories stimulating fat storage but also by simulating the effects of hormones on your cells, slowing your metabolism, and promoting fat production. They also affect the genetic code. It has less to do with your carbohydrate or fat intake and more to do with the entire combination of exposures you have.

The DNA in your body is modified, activating survival genes to make things happen out of control. Weight gain and uncontrolled cell division and growth of cancer are examples. We fight genetics but not as we once thought. Genes are modified on multiple levels from many stimuli. Cells in your body react when they are exposed to light, temperature, nutrients, hormones, oxygen, free radicals, toxins, and radiation. Each modifies the activation or inactivation of certain genes to give you the unique combination that determines who you will be. The exposures shape the subtle difference in your facial features, the variation of eye color within your family, and the difference in how you laugh. These stimuli can affect behavior as well.

But it gets worse, or better, depending on your point of view. Genetic material is modified in every cell, and this includes the gametes or reproductive cells within the ovaries and testicles. The DNA of every potential child can be affected. Is the incidence of cancer increasing? Yup. Is the incidence of diabetes increasing? Yup. Is the incidence of obesity increasing? Yup. Is the incidence of behavioral problems increasing? Yup. Children are being born with their genes activated to be fat, sick, hyperactive, autistic, and ready to die.

Why does nature allow this? It's actually a clever survival mechanism that has been sabotaged. It makes a lot of sense from a survival standpoint, to be able to activate or inactivate certain survival genes as needed. For example, fever might help you get over an infection but it would be problematic if you were feverish all the time. But think about the impact this might have on a person living in nature. If the parents live in an environment that is stressful or lacks certain nutrients, it makes sense that the unborn child is prepared to survive in that environment. The parents' environment and behavior activate or inactivate certain genes to give the child a survival advantage as soon as they are born.

Imagine a mother living in a desert area where food is scarce and there is little water and nutrition. A child born with the genes activated to slow metabolism and save fat definitely has the survival advantage. People who live in desert regions want genes that deal with excess heat and saving water to be activated. It also makes sense that their children are born with the same characteristics so that they can survive the environment they are coming into. Similar adaptations happen with cold and other challenges like the lack of nutrition. Not having enough nutrition can actually stress the body and set off weight gain. Infants born to parents who live in such an environment are already primed to take on the same characteristics of weight gain as the parents, only more so.

Any environmental stimulus has the potential to cause gene modification. This can be from what we eat, nutrients, drink, or toxins. Substances inhaled from the air can do this as well, like smoking or other pollution. As more research reveals how genes are modified, we see why simple diet and exercise may not be effective in changing obesity. So many things have an impact on how your genes are expressed, like intensity of sunlight, exposure to artificial light, ambient temperature, and social interactions. Surprising, right? These components stimulate the perpetual fall and directly modify your genes.

Why the obsession with weight? Why not talk about other genes and diseases? Many illnesses, diseases, conditions, ailments, and problems arise from obesity. Weight is the symbol of a greater problem and condition. Our disconnection with the natural cycles and processes that other animals participate in has led to a plethora of evolving problems. By eating what we were not intended to eat, drinking what we were not intended to drink, breathing what we were not intended to breathe, and living where we were not intended to live, we have led ourselves down the road to disaster. It is important to realize the path we are on is unhealthy and return to a better path to health.

How much can this make a difference? What can eating better and losing excess body fat do for us? The stories about the transformative effect on people's health are plentiful. Diabetes can be reversed or improved. Heart disease risk can be decreased. Even severe disease such as metastatic ovarian cancer spread throughout the body, usually fatal and untreatable with conventional methods, can be reversed by a dramatic change in lifestyle (Oshakbayev, 2014). There is always hope for everyone to make a change in their life and health, and always a way to avoid or fight the cats that assault our genes every day.

Everything begins with the triggers (cats) in your life. Once you know these, the question to ask yourself is, "Do I want to leave myself at the mercy of a room full of cats?" Instead of allowing the environment to modify you, choose what you eat and drink, and your environment wisely. Choose what you see and hear, and who you spend time with. Instead of allowing change to happen, be your own agent of change. Be the CAT. Learn the language of your cells and DNA and tell them to give up the fat for good!

Signs of Spring

Spring is immortalized in songs, paintings, poems, and our general psyche. It signals a turn from the hardship and scarcity, confinement and worry of winter to rebirth. Easter fits with the ancient rites celebrating the "death" of earth in winter and rebirth with new life in spring. Animals reappear, plants send out leaves, and the world is lit with brighter sunlight. These events and changes stimulate activity, increase metabolism and wakefulness, improve healing, and reduce the winter depression people languish in during the darker months.

More nutrients are available in early spring and summer versus fall. Such fruits as raspberries flower in late spring and produce fruit early in summer. They keep us active by allowing the use of stored energy more efficiently. This is particularly important for an animal that has weathered the winter and waits for most of the food to appear. Raspberry ketones increase lipolysis (breakdown of fat), even with high fat diets (Park, 2010). Ketones signal your body to release that last bit of stored energy from winter so you can hunt for new food sources and rebuild what was lost in muscle mass. Without these kinds of signals, your fat storing genes remain active.

Fat stores continue to diminish during the spring even while you start to put on muscle. But raspberries are not the only fat burning fruit or vegetable. Others are just as effective but not as glamorous. Some combinations of foods or substances have a greater fat burning effect than any one by itself (Murosaki, 2007). Choose the nutrition you need to maximize the benefits of your overall diet. Don't get stuck eating the same foods all year. The variety from seasonality and eating food that is local and fresh guarantees you get the right amounts of fat burning substances when they are needed.

How do phytochemicals, or plant-derived substances, affect your fat loss? There are three suspected mechanisms. While these have yet to be proven, there is good evidence all three may be working.

Frequently, manufacturers attempt to bottle phytochemicals. The problem is when you extract the "fat burning substance" from food you lose much of what it was supposed to do. Instead of water, sugars, fiber, and vitamins you have an isolated chemical that may not function well outside of its natural source. More importantly, you gain potential toxicity from the substance when concentrated. Every week on a health TV show or weight loss website is talk about the latest jungle fruit that magically reduces your waistline. No magic pill, potion, or berries will get you to slim down. There are significant long-term costs and complications from these quick fixes and they don't work for everyone. That is why you hear about a great cure one day and it disappears from the news a few weeks later. Marketers use your desire for a convenient answer or cure. They sell you a "fat burner" with little benefit without telling you it doesn't work for everyone, and as soon as you stop taking it and return to old habits the weight will be back.

Over twenty well-studied phytochemicals (chemicals from plants) contribute to weight loss, with thousands more that have yet to be researched. While these work individually, they are better in combinations. That's why eating the same fruit or vegetable all the time isn't as effective as having some variety. The phytochemicals work by three different mechanisms to help with weight loss:

1. Decreasing the number of stem cells that will turn into fat cells (adipocyte stem cells)
2. Increased apoptosis (programmed cell death) of fat cells (adipocytes)
3. Blocking dietary fat absorption

The more vegetables and fruits you get, the better. You want food when its substances are in the highest concentration. This happens when they're most flavorful, and have the strongest scent and most color—when the fruit or vegetable is ripe in season. Not every fruit is the best option for weight loss though. It is important to recognize another characteristic that many of us have never dealt with.

Glycemic index will soon be a household concern. Certain foods can raise your blood sugar very high and others have less of an impact. Higher sugar levels cause insulin secretion, which drives fat storage. By looking at the impact foods have on your blood sugar level, you can successfully balance your sugar levels to prevent peaks and troughs throughout the day. These high glycemic foods lead to high insulin and glucagon release causing weight gain and uncontrolled hunger. Low glycemic foods can help to stop the cycle of fat storage and weight gain, but even healthy foods can be sabotaged. Foods in combination eaten at different times have a different impact on blood sugar. For example, a bowl of healthy steel cut oatmeal and a glass of orange juice on the side is a high glycemic meal that adds more weight. Simply switch the juice to a whole orange and the benefits are regained.

Include the fruits and vegetables of spring and leave out the starchy fall vegetables and processed grains. Eating only what is available in spring will have a drastic impact on your blood sugar and total calorie intake. Fruits and vegetables contain carbohydrates. Stick with those in season and start your day with a vegetable or low-glycemic fruit. Eating berries that ripen in spring and early summer gives you great fat burning phytochemicals, vitamins, and minerals, and protect you from another group of fat-gaining substances. They help reduce the formation of advanced glycation end-products (AGEs). These come from excess sugars, refined starches, and overcooking, and put you at risk for heart disease, aging, Alzheimer's, and weight gain. Berries also reduce appetite when taken as a snack between meals. Taking the right foods at the right time of year helps you achieve great health improvements.

You can also time when you eat carbohydrates through the day. This concept is called "carb-cycling." You've been told carbohydrates are bad, but there are no bad nutrients. Carbohydrates, fat, and protein are all important. There's not one culprit for weight gain. It's a process with multiple factors and more related to the lack of micronutrients and the timing of the macronutrients. Carbohydrates and glycemic index are responsible for some weight gain. Now, many nutrition experts and exercise professionals are promoting carb-cycling. You take higher amounts of carbohydrates at certain times and lower amounts at other times to achieve a higher level of weight loss and muscle gain than with a low carbohydrate diet.

You may have heard about the benefits of eating carbohydrates in the morning, before exercise, or after exercise. Each of us is a little different. People who are diabetic notice their blood sugars higher in the morning so this means morning isn't for everyone. Before exercise is a good idea if you plan a heavy workout and worry about fatigue. If you haven't shifted to a healthier diet, you probably don't need to do this, but focus on adding better options. Carbohydrate and protein intake should be four hours before a workout to make it beneficial.

Athletes can use carb-cycling to optimize muscle and strength gains and improve performance. For the average person interested in fat loss and improving your health, there is a better way. Do this only when you are committed to preparing or planning meals ahead of time. Delaying carbohydrates for two hours after exercise leaves your muscle glycogen depleted. The only way your body can replenish this is to start accessing your fat stores. Your weight loss will be much more efficient without resorting to complex timing strategies on what foods to eat.

How about after exercise for the average person? Take a good source of protein and healthy carbohydrate, like a protein shake and piece of fruit. Is this the most efficient way to lose fat? Used in conjunction with exercise, they can be very effective. Why? The majority of people don't plan their meals in advance. When they finish exercising, they're hungry and will gravitate to the most convenient food to fill their rumbling bellies and replenish their drained energy stores. This can frequently be fast food or other unhealthy options. Taking a healthy choice right after working out encourages muscle gain, rewards you for the positive activity, and satisfies you long enough to prepare a healthy meal. Protein, fat, and carbs are all important after exercise, but they have to be healthy types and in the right proportions to encourage muscle building and replenish glycogen without storing fat.

Protein shakes count as processed foods and, in general, I advise against reliance on them but there is rarely a one hundred percent rule. Having a healthy source of convenient protein will help make the transition to healthy eating easier. A high quality meal replacement or protein supplement is a better option when you are in a hurry or very hungry and definitely better than fast food. The problem is that many meal replacements substitute healthy decisions for taste, marketing, or packaging concerns. It's important to make sure that it's a high quality supplement and that you actually know what type of protein you are getting. This is because the type of protein makes a difference in its benefit for weight loss too. A natural protein found in spring is the milk protein, whey. Most of us don't get enough nutrition to support muscle growth from exercise and eating enough may come with too much extra fat or carbs and may not be practical. That's where these protein supplements may come in.

Modern farming and cattle breeding produces calves and milk all year. In nature, spring is the calving season and the start of new milk production. Supplementing with whey is important for stimulating muscle growth and decreasing muscle loss when restricting calories (Hector, 2015). One study demonstrated over twenty-one percent greater weight loss over a thirteen-week period while it stopped muscle loss (Verreijen, 2015). How much should you take? Your total protein intake should be 0.08 to 0.1 ounces per pound (1 to 1.5 grams per kilogram) of body weight per day. Athletes may need more to support big muscle gains. Some people advocate more, but there's not sufficient evidence for this in all people.

Not everyone will lose excess weight by adding milk protein to their diet, since some people have sensitivities that eliminate it as an option. Others have renal disease making it less desirable and making plant proteins and other sources better options such as in the Paleolithic diet. The Paleolithic diet is where processed carbohydrates and many modern foods are eliminated in favor of what you catch, hunt, or gather. The idea is that if you have less processed foods and substitute more natural foods you can reduce weight gain. This actually works, but there is more to it than the oversimplification of a "diet." The Paleolithic diet is a lifestyle, and following its precepts and building good habits lead to success. We tend to oversimplify the concept of eating naturally sometimes and forget what is needed.

The Paleolithic diet has a missing component. Paleolithic people didn't fish, gather, or capture the same things all year. In fact, they often saw things for a limited time and not again until the following year. The seasons of food were extremely important. Seasonal abundance and saturation with certain nutrients happened when those nutrients were needed. When Paleolithic people came across a tree with fruit on its branches, they ate their fill and possibly collected some for later. If the tree were close enough to their home range, they returned for several days for more fruit. They would eat almost to the exclusion of other foods except the fruits that were also in season. We rarely do this today. Most foods are available all year and even then, we rarely eat a large quantity of one food.

People with seasonal gardens are familiar with this. When they finish the last squash, they don't want squash again for the whole year. Substitute in any vegetable or fruit you grow and you've likely had your fill by the end of the season. How many of us eat bananas all year? When Thanksgiving leftovers are finally finished, you don't want to see another turkey or cranberry until next Thanksgiving. If you had to eat all the bananas you normally consume annually in a two-month period, would you have bananas again? This is often the case in Third World countries. Fruits and vegetables are available in their season and then gone. By the time you finish that last, black, overripe banana you can't stand another one.

Eat Seasonal, Eat Fresh

A good diet is more than getting protein, eating low glycemic, and taking vitamins. You may have heard about "getting your five a day," eating three vegetables and two fruits per day as the minimum needed to maintain a healthy weight and good macronutrient content. This seems obvious but most people in the U.S. and around the world don't understand this (Guenther, 2006). In fact, recommendations for the number of servings are higher (some say six to ten, others say higher) but it's already difficult to convince people to eat just the five a day.

It's like surfing without having been on a surfboard. You might find it easier if you practice balancing or paddling the board out. Similarly, eating six to ten vegetables and fruits sounds like you need to camp in the middle of a field and eat all day long. It's easier once you get started and practice. Estimates vary but U.S. government sites and many media outlets claim that only 27.4 percent of people get their three vegetables per day. Only 32.8 percent get their two fruits, and only fourteen percent of Americans eat all five. The numbers vary depending on where you look. The point is we are far short of where we should be.

Are you part of the 67.2 percent that don't eat enough fruits and vegetables? Keep track with a food intake journal as suggested in *Fast-Track Your Health*. I periodically do this as a reality check so I can do better. The journal makes you accountable for getting what you need, like supplements for the nutrients you miss. Changing your health, losing weight, and shutting off your fat gene demands you take action on a regular basis. You can do this in a healthy way.

Eating in Season

A mango out of season is usually hard and green. Cut into one and it has a sour, pasty flavor that coats your tongue and makes you dread the next mango. You can leave it out on the counter, wrap it in newspapers, put it in a ripening bag, bury it in sand, or any number of tricks to encourage the mango to ripen. The problem is that the fruit never ripens properly because it was picked before its natural time in order to increase its shipping and shelf life. Usually these mangoes sit on the counter or in the fridge until they are wrinkled, covered with brown spots and more inedible than when they were unripe.

Now contrast that with a tree ripened fruit.

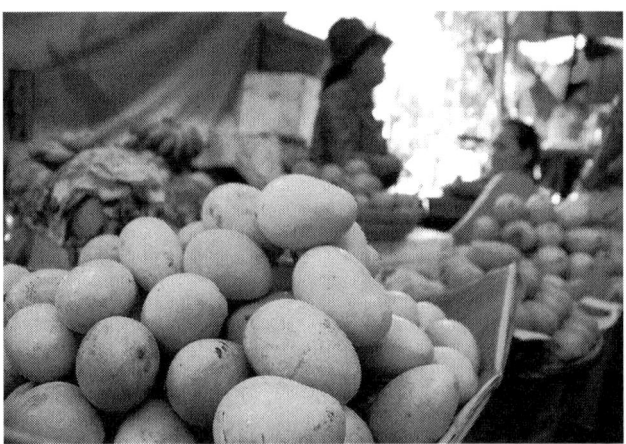

A fresh off the tree ripe fruit smells and tastes amazing. You can't get enough. It's common for children in places with fresh fruit to eat until they are sick. My family did it with wild blackberries when I was younger in Houston, and mangoes and oranges in Miami. We ate mulberries when living in Connecticut until our lips and fingers were stained purple and we were sick from eating too much. While visiting family in Pennsylvania, I remember ripe white-fleshed peaches the size of softballs. They smelled amazing and tasted as sweet as honey. You had to lean forward to keep the juice from running down your chin and on your shirt. The orchard let us eat as many as we wanted as we picked them to buy. I thought I could eat a dozen but after the second one, my stomach was so full I could hardly breathe. Each region and country has local fruits at their peak and greatest abundance during a certain time of year. There may be a second crop but it is never the same as the main season.

The convention of four distinct seasons is not everywhere. Some parts of the country or world have only two seasons and others have variations in weather without distinct seasons. Eating fruits and vegetables at the right time is very important. We are just learning the value of what foods contain at different times of the year. Each food contains different nutrients essential to your health. The variety and timing of food is key. Native plants in certain areas give a health advantage over non-native foods.

For instance, I'm from Texas and Texas has many edible native plants with significant nutritional value. Many of these plants were eaten by native peoples and provided necessary nutrients besides calories. The advantages go beyond availability and convenience. Those plants adapted to the local environment over millennia with substances that allowed them to better survive. Evidence shows that you can gain health advantages by eating those foods (Pan et al., 2013). Hold on, I'm not suggesting you go into your backyard and start chowing down on the weeds (although some have more nutrition than typical salad contents), but our palate of fruits and vegetables has become very small and monotonous. It also includes foods from regions with different climates than where you live.

There is definitely a role for seeing more of certain nutrients at certain times of the year, like the appropriate antioxidants. This helps reduce the risk of heart disease when it's greatest or when cholesterol levels are naturally higher. We know that risk of certain conditions changes at different times of the year, such as winter. For example, metabolic syndrome is a condition when you have three of the following: fat storage around the abdomen, elevated blood pressure, elevated fasting blood glucose level, high serum triglycerides, and low high-density lipoprotein (HDL)/good cholesterol levels. This puts you in danger of diabetes and heart disease. Metabolic syndrome is more common in winter than summer. The difference in prevalence can be as much as five percent higher (Kamezaki, 2010). Your cholesterol level can be as much as sixteen percent higher in winter and vitamin C levels can drop sixteen percent in the winter months.

The flavor of fruits will change with the seasons. The thirty-one compounds that give strawberries their flavor change in quantity over time and not by the same amount. This means an almost infinite variability in the quality of flavor and scents of strawberries. These correlate with the location, weather, sunlight, nutrients, and the soil and water (Schwieterman, 2014). The same variations in nutrients and flavor occur in every plant. It's not just about flavor, though. These nutrients are chemicals made by the plants (or "phytonutrients") and can have significant impacts on our health. For instance, phytonutrients in cherries can help us overcome joint pains and improve diabetes (Bell et al., 2014; Lachin, 2014). It's important to get the fruits and vegetables when they have the peak of these useful substances for our health.

Eating seasonally means eating plenty of fresh vegetables, fruits, grains, and meats appearing at that time of year. Variation in the diet as well as abundance (in nutrients, not over-eating) gives your body the nutritional and seasonal signals to allow weight loss. When you limit your calorie intake, the body compensates by slowing metabolism. You can do the same work using less energy. This is like trading in your regular car for a hybrid. It's the same car, but gets better mileage on the same fuel. Studies have demonstrated people that eat very little, often less than they need based on their weight and activity, will continue to gain weight. Part of this is by better energy extraction through gut flora and higher efficiency in energy use.

Slowed metabolism and increased body efficiency is why many weight loss attempts including weight loss surgeries are doomed to fail. The drastic reduction in calories and nutrition may lead to a temporary drop in weight, but the body's ability to modify the metabolic rate make this unsustainable. Good evidence shows that most people can tolerate a fifteen percent calorie deficit during heavy physical activity and maintain their weight due to the metabolic rate regulating energy use. By keeping the metabolic rate active, you lose weight in a healthy and sustainable fashion. Careful planning will save you from trying to restart your metabolism, which is harder than keeping it running.

Food deserts are areas in cities where there is no access to nutritive foods. Foods swamps are areas where fatty or unhealthy processed foods outnumber healthier choices. Both of these are becoming common in the U.S. and are beginning to occur worldwide. The scarcity of fresh, healthy alternatives makes it challenging to maintain good eating habits that give essential nutrients. By allowing nutrient scarcity, we are setting ourselves up for the perpetual fall. Efforts by many courageous people are trying to change this desert and swamp distribution of food by bringing fresh foods and markets to inner cities.

Processed foods are considered a luxury in many countries. Many people have switched to unhealthy processed foods to show how successful they are. They spend the fruits of their labor avoiding real fruits only to pay later when told to eat fruit. This vicious cycle is seen in many developing countries. Brazil is a good example (Ferolla, 2013). Recommendations for healthy eating are considered "low class" or out of touch. In a few years when obesity starts to take the lives of their families and steal their health, they will be in the same situation as people in the U.S. Getting back to eating the natural healthy fruits and vegetables is a key first step.

Some fruits and vegetables have a single growing season where they flower and produce. Others may have two growing cycles and two harvests. The light, water, temperature, and other conditions are different for both harvests. A spring harvest of one vegetable may be different in nutrient content from the fall. The demand for certain fruits and vegetables year round has forced producers to get them from other regions or grow them in climates or countries that are not native. This gives the fruits and vegetables different characteristics. Wine aficionados know that the region grapes are grown in and the weather during a particular year are just as important as the variety of the grape. The environment the grapes were grown in determines the flavor and nutrients they contain. The same goes for any other fruit or vegetable, although we don't have asparagus tastings or broccoli tours.

Even meat is seasonal. We eat Thanksgiving turkey and the Christmas goose because that's when these animals were hunted, and were their fattest and most plentiful. Fish have a season. The annual running of the salmon or migration of sardines prompted seasonal eating of these fish. Many countries have traditions stemming from the seasonal appearance of animals and plants in their region. Festivals, celebrations, and feasts are built around what is plentiful at certain times of the year. Animals growing, gaining weight, and bearing young are factors in the seasons when they are vulnerable, tasty, and easily hunted.

Look up "cherry festival" or "strawberry festival" online and you will find tons of information. Substitute any fruit, vegetable, or meat for similar results. These events happen when the food item is most available. People have so much of a particular food at this time of year that they want new and creative ways to eat it—pies, jellies, fried, baked, and stuffed. Each seasonal food item is spiced to make it more palatable when in excess, or preserved for when it's less plentiful.

A benefit of eating in season is "seasonal saturation," where you get an overabundance of a particular nutrient. When fruits, vegetables, grains, and meats only appeared in a certain time of year, you had a limited opportunity to eat a large quantity. You would get a lot of the same nutrient in a short time. Detox or cleansing means ridding yourself of the accumulated toxins that build up throughout the year or your lifetime. The repair and reversal of damage by eating an abundance of antioxidant rich foods happens this way. An example of this seasonal saturation is the appearance of citrus fruits in the fall and early winter. They provide an abundance of vitamin C that helps to counteract the rise of cholesterol that will be coming in winter.

Seasonal foods are only there for a short period of time, so you have no choice but to eat what is available. There are also a much greater variety of foods available, greens, fruits, vegetables, grains, and meats we don't consider food any more. Most of us have spent more than one Saturday and Sunday, not to mention money and intense labor, getting rid of "weeds" that a few generations ago were key staples in our diet. We destroy what used to keep our ancestors alive and healthy.

Seasonal saturation is counterbalanced by "seasonal scarcity," the times of the year with little of this same nutrient. This helps to set your internal clock through a complex series of metabolic processes (Wu, 2015) and reduces the negative impact of any particular food or toxin throughout the year. Seasonality isn't the only clock at work. The internal clocks of animals are important to their weight loss or gain and their efficient use of nutrients, but plants have an internal clock as well.

Plants are thought of as passive green objects that only move in the wind, but they are fully alive and capable of defending themselves against attack. They alter the substances within to resist sunlight and other environmental challenges. Plants also produce defensive substances. Insects are a major challenge to any plant. Those who have no substances to defend themselves disappear very quickly. Insects have a daily cycle of eating—some feeding earlier in the day and others later. The plants these insects feed on have developed a cycle of producing substances to fend off attacks (Pare, 1999). They do this at the right time of day. It doesn't make sense to spend energy to defend yourself all day long if you only get attacked in the morning.

The substances are stimulated by a natural cycle of exposure to sunlight at certain times, for certain lengths, and with certain nutrients present. Like you, their internal clock and sun exposure, as well as other environmental signals, determine what happens inside. Without these factors, the plants become helpless to defend themselves and rely on us to spray them with pesticides. These chemical pesticides will also contribute to weight gain.

Many of a plant's defenses, known as phytochemicals, give us health benefits as well: anticancer, anti-aging, and even anti-obesity effects (Zhang, 2015). Sustainable farming practices maintain these benefits in the plants we rely on for food. Eliminating chemical fertilizers and pesticides preserves the environment and your health, and reduces the cost of healthcare. Most important, you enjoy your life more since you are healthier. This brings up the inevitable question, "How much does eating healthy cost?"

Cheap is Never Cheap

There is a common belief that eating healthy is expensive, but this is a myth promoted by the fast food and processed food industries, as well as an excuse for people who know what they should do, but haven't done. It's easier to have a reason and excuse than take on the unfamiliar and get the results you want. Research has shown eating unhealthy costs more. For example, it takes sixty-one cents to super-size a meal. This translates into over six dollars in extra cost for healthcare, and extra fuel to move around the extra weight you put on.

Grapes in season can be as cheap as $2.98 for a three-pound box. The same grapes in January cost over seven dollars, more than double than when in season. My local grocery store chain finally realized the cost obesity had on its own bottom line because it paid out more on employee benefits for healthcare and insurance. This, plus a sense of social responsibility, led them to hire a full-time dietitian and organize nutrition classes and grocery store tours. They also showed comparisons of how far your money goes when you purchase unhealthy versus healthy foods.

Here is an example of how far your money goes. Twenty dollars is not much when you walk into the grocery store, but look at how it can be used: one way is to eat "healthy," the second is "easy" or convenient, and the last is "cheap." I call it "cheap" because most people will spend money on a movie, soda, or coffee but they agonize over an extra dollar or two on a healthy food item. It's like they don't deserve it. For twenty dollars you can get:

"Healthy"	"Easy"	"Cheap"
1 pound lean ground turkey $3.47	1 large Dominos specialty pizza $15.99	Honeynut Cheerios $4.70
2 pounds dried black beans $2.89	2 liter Coke $2.49	1 gallon 1% milk $2.70
1 pound strawberries $1.94		Hot pockets $9.98
1 bunch broccoli $1.65		Tropicana 64oz orange juice $3.98
1 pound spinach $1.65		
2 pounds bananas $0.99		
2 medium onions $0.98		
1 head garlic $0.58		
1/2 pound steel cut oats $2.86		
2 green bell pepper $1.36		
1 red bell pepper $0.78		
3 cans tomato sauce $1.00	+ tax	
Total: $20.15	**$20.21**	**$21.36**

You get more nutritious and overall volume of food when you buy healthy. You may get more carbohydrates and calories eating "cheap" or "easy," but who wants to be cheap, easy, and overweight? The healthy option has more vitamins, minerals, water, fiber, and protein. This is just one example but you can repeat this and your grocery basket will always fill up with more food, especially when you pay attention to specials on produce and meat.

Even if it were expensive to eat healthy, or only organic foods, this is an investment in your health. Pay the money now to enjoy nutritious food that allows you to lose and maintain your weight, or pay a drug company, doctor, or hospital later to treat the resulting illnesses. Paying a little extra now means you can travel and play into your later years. Giving up a few dollars today will make sure your body looks thirty when you're fifty or sixty. Hundreds of inspirational videos on the Internet show people making dramatic personal transformations in their health or weight. Usually it comes after a health scare or they are fed up with not getting better with healthcare. "Healthcare" is an inaccurate term because what most doctors and hospitals do is disease treatment after your health has been lost. Why put yourself through being unable to walk, severe heart disease, and diabetes? Start prevention now.

Many of us are willing to spend four to five dollars per day on coffee, yet hesitate to shop healthy. What else do you spend your time and money on that doesn't help or has a negative impact on your health? A two-hour movie with popcorn and soda costs twenty or more dollars and you still wonder why you can't afford to eat well. Going to a restaurant costs thirty or forty dollars, and you can't afford supplements you need. The resources are there. Improvement in your health, appearance, and energy level may lead you to new opportunities that bring you to even more resources. This is basic human psychology and biology. All animals gauge the health of the members of their species and much of it is based on behavior and appearance. Humans are no different. In fact, we create artificial criteria to classify each other as okay or inferior based on clothing and hairstyle. Don't be surprised that your appearance, energy level, and weight place you in a category you don't want to be in or cause people to prejudge you. The real question is, how do you view yourself? Are you worth spending on you and your family to be healthier? The answer is obviously yes.

Your personal commitment to eating healthy will be seen by others as a respect for yourself and they will in turn give you respect. Being educated about what you buy and eat is an investment in good health. Spend the four to five dollars for your daily coffee toward your health for a couple of months and you will see significant improvements, and have the energy to no longer need coffee. Have you ever said, "I *need* my coffee?" Substitute any random drug name into that sentence and say it with the same passion and emotion. Just imagine saying, "I *need* my cocaine" or "I *need* my heroin." Pretty silly, right? This illustrates that a great deal of emphasis is placed on something that shouldn't be important and has no positive impact in your health. You would never consider alcohol or drugs to cope with personal problems, yet accept caffeine as a good solution for fatigue.

What else do you spend money on to cover symptoms of nutritional deficiencies? Start fixing the underlying problems by selecting good food and knowing where your food comes from. Only about eighteen cents of every dollar you spend on food is spent on growing it. The rest goes to shipping, marketing, storage, and packaging. Having a relationship with local farmers and friends with gardens is a great way to be sure you know where the food came from. You also get more for your dollar. This isn't always possible, but even having friends who plant things that are complimentary to your garden ensures freshness and variety. Having your own garden and developing these relationships will give you good food, sun, exercise, and a support network that can help you get the best results in life.

Personal commitments and decisions are important because labels such as natural, organic, non-GMO, and healthy don't guarantee what you are getting is actually good for you. Go to your local farmer's market and get to know people. Talk, ask questions, and be involved with your food. Having a relationship with the people who produce your food will help your health. Choose to invest in your health with fresh, healthy, local produce and meats from people you know who care about you and your family. Save money and be healthy while eating seasonal and fresh.

The Fat Foods of Fall

Fall foods are, in general, those that appear when the weather is shifting from the hottest to cooling again. Since "Fall" or autumn is not a universal season it is better to think of the transition from long to short days and heat to cooler temperatures. Those of you who are older still remember a time when you would only see apples in the late summer and fall. Apple festivals and apple picking are still held in many places in the country in the fall, yet apples are in stores all year. Oranges were also linked to the fall or winter. Remember the song, "Chestnuts Roasting on an Open Fire"? There is a reason why such songs remain a part of our culture. These foods were only available at certain times of the year. They were abundant and after we had our fill, we didn't see them again for a full year. Many of these foods were combined to give us the fall diet.

What is the fall diet? In the United States, think of a traditional Thanksgiving dinner. This will give you a good idea of the fall diet. The foods at that time of year were very important for survival back in the Pilgrim days and why they are so important in our culture— that critical link to survival of the people who founded the country. Over time, the actual foods have changed slightly and how we got those foods shifted dramatically. It's not just the actual foods. It's more the combination of nutrients and lack of certain key nutrients that creates the fall diet. A preponderance of sugars, starches, fatty meats, fall vegetables, and fall fruits triggers your internal clock to read, "fall." Once set to fall, you are primed to gain weight just like animals during that time of year. You are programmed to eat more and store more fat in response to those signals.

People tend to combine starches and fats in the fall, like mashed potatoes and dinner rolls with butter. Adding sugary sides such as cranberry sauce next to fatty meats and other dishes continues the combination. Even green bean casserole, something you think of as healthy, combines fat and starches to drive weight gain. Think of the desserts that often come after the meal. Pies and cookies have a combination of carbohydrates and fat that are sure to send anyone's blood sugar skyrocketing and drive fat to be stored where you least want it.

Combining these foods drives a vicious up and down cycle in blood sugar. This can drive overeating, leading to high blood sugar, or hyperglycemia, and cause sudden insulin release driving your blood sugar way down. The sugar goes down by being taken into the cells of your body and stored as fat. When you have low blood sugar, your body protects itself by releasing epinephrine, cortisol, and glucagon leading to more overeating. This causes a repeat of the process and leads to a fat gain rollercoaster. You may have experienced this as the so-called food coma after Thanksgiving dinner where everyone's asleep on the couch and then back in the kitchen eating again in 30 minutes.

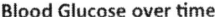

Blood Glucose over time

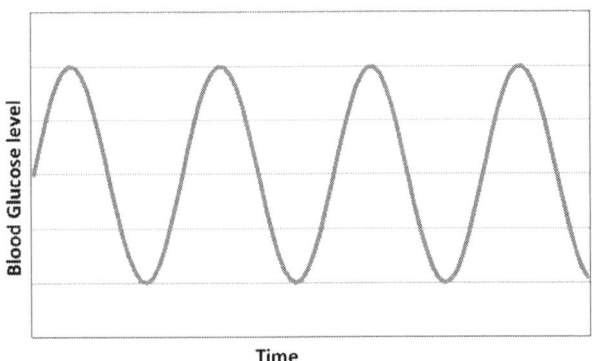

Nutrients in Fall

Subtle differences in the nutrient content of foods that appear in the fall help signal your body it is time to gain or release fat. There is also a specific trigger to eat more. Fat in your diet is extremely important, but for now, I'll focus on the other nutrients in food and how these differ at different times of year. Many people have talked about the obvious: overeating, too many carbohydrates, too much or the wrong types of fat in the diet. Everyone is subject to how the body uses these nutrients and will determine if you store or release fat. Fat is stored or used as energy depending not only on your metabolism and activity but also on having the right enzymes and hormones to break down the fat. Without the appropriate function of your enzymes and hormones, you can't use the fat and carbohydrates effectively as energy and end up storing them. It's not just specific foods, but how nutrients are presented or prepared that makes a difference.

What determines enzyme function includes the micronutrients that come from food. If the food—meat, grains, vegetables, or fruits—lacks appropriate micronutrients, you will have a problem. Unfortunately, how, when, and where the food is produced is just as important as what type of food you eat. Nutrient content has changed over time and we are frequently deficient in key nutrients we no longer get in our food.

Certain vegetables often produced two crops, a spring or summer and a fall or winter crop. The characteristics of the foods from two seasons are different in their nutrient content and provide different benefits during the year. The level of antioxidants and other key nutrients vary between months during the same harvesting season (Zhang, 2013). It is important to know if you actually benefit from the foods you eat and if they are as healthy as you think. It is even more important when you consider we now eat them all year. Foods are available from distant geographic locations and seasonal extremes when we used to see them for only limited times during the year. What we have done with introduction of foods from other locations is introduce nutrients at wrong times, allow toxins to persist all year, and further disconnect ourselves from the natural cycle. This limits the nutrients you would normally absorb.

The globalization and industrialization of world markets and the demand for certain items out-of-season has driven the availability of many foods outside of their natural season. One side effect of all-year food availability is that people no longer crave the foods they did in the past. We haven't experienced the variety and flavor that nature seasonally provides. Cravings are blunted when you see foods through the year. Because you never see a burst of certain nutrients, you don't know the difference between having a lot and having a little. Instead, nutrients come in a trickle that never truly replenishes your stores of vitamins and minerals but instead allows you to become deficient slowly over time.

The all-year availability of foods also creates the sense that "I can pick the foods I like at any time." Unfortunately, thousands of years of evolution have programmed you to like the tastes of certain types of foods and less than a hundred years of marketing and fast food has taken advantage of these tastes. What happens is you repeatedly eat the same foods hoping they will provide you with the nutrients you need when you know they won't. Cravings happen and you can never satisfy them. We no longer know what our body needs. Nutrients previously contained in foods became separated and removed with modern processing and farming. This leaves behind the bad while taking out the good. The awareness of this and how to add back in nutrition is important. Let's look at what drives you to prefer certain foods and perpetuate these problems. After all, we can't change farming practices, marketing, or modern food manufacturing overnight. You have to find what you can do for your own health to defend against outside forces.

Fall and winter vegetables have a sweeter flavor compared to the spring and summer. This is due to a difference in the substances produced by the plants during these times of year. Plants have to protect themselves more from pests in spring and summer, and produce substances to repel them at those times. They also need protection from sunlight and produce pigments to do just that. We often prefer the fall crop due to the sweeter flavor and drive demand from other parts of the world. Unfortunately, we eat fewer of the spring and summer vegetables because of their bitter flavor. We are programmed to deal with the difference in seasonal flavors of produce (Ileri-Gurel, 2013). When temperature changes to cold, your threshold for detecting sweet and salty flavors goes up meaning you need more sweet or salty to get the same flavor (Al'Absi, 2012). Stress in general, whether from temperature or other sources, modulates your taste through the stress hormone cortisol, which helps control sugar and salt metabolism.

Taste preferences drive the demand for sweeter foods. The demand and the commoditization of our food supply have eliminated the normal variety and seasonal variation once seen in the food supply. Variation and variety used to be the sign of a good farmer. Native Americans and many other traditional cultures knew this and planted accordingly. Several crops were planted in the same field, or rotated annually. This protected the plants from pests, gave higher yields, and guaranteed sustainability. Output and homogeneity has become the new standard by which we judge farm success. This homogeneity has been good for agribusiness bottom lines but has created a huge problem in nutrition, health, and buying habits. It has driven many farms and farmers out of business and created an environmental problem that was unanticipated.

Monoculture Farming

Farms that produce only a single crop, or monoculture, are susceptible to any blight, disease, or pest attracted to that crop. The farms also are subject to any price fluctuation on that crop. You have heard about diversification when it comes to an investment portfolio and this applies to the farming industry. It is no wonder that we get the term "don't put your eggs in one basket" from farmers as a warning not to put all your hopes on one crop lest it fail or be destroyed. Relying on monoculture has been no boon to small farmers. Farmers who try to compete against agricultural corporations face the problems of scale economy in that the larger producer is able to produce more for less or pay less to its suppliers—the farmers. This has resulted in regionalization of many of our crops in America. Large swathes of corn, wheat, and soybean crops are subject to the same environmental and economic risks. When they are in one area, one bad rainy season or dry season can potentially destroy the entire crop or affect prices, world markets, and eating habits.

Giant monoculture farms also have other major problems. Bees and insects help pollinate flowers and are the farmer's friends when it comes to boosting outputs. Monoculture farming creates a huge opportunity for bees and insects in one short season of flowering. This is like setting up a temporary all-you-can-eat buffet with only one item, leaving them to starve for the rest of the year. Having crop variety by region not only makes sense for consumers but also for the farmer as a hedge on seasonal crop markets and climate impacts. More importantly, it helps to maintain the insect ecosystem that in turn feeds into the larger food web we are a part of.

Unfortunately we also spray all kinds of chemicals onto our food to protect them from the insects. This may kill the good along with the bad leading to a cascade of problems. These pesticides and other substances sprayed on the plants can leave residues or be absorbed into the plant, fruit, or vegetable. This passes on to us! We are just beginning to unravel the effects of this toxic cocktail on our health and weight. Plant variety on a farm is a way to naturally diversify the insects and also to potentially protect more sensitive plants.

We have failed to recognize that many of the insects are essential for long-term crop production and sustainability. With monoculture, there is more incentive to protect that crop from harmful pests using pesticides. These harmful residues on food can mimic hormones promoting fat storage and have other harmful side effects. It can reduce crop production and lead to the need for genetic manipulation to get the same yield without the aid of the insects.

Another major drawback of monoculture farming practice is there is so much riding on one crop that the producers are compelled to find more ways to present it to us. By altering flavors, packaging, and marketing, you see the same products again, only disguised. Like painting your car, it looks pretty but is still the same car under the paint. Imagine being given nothing but corn to eat every meal, every day, and every week for a month. How would you feel after one day? After two days? Now imagine the whole month. You probably would stop eating and be starving, sick, and never want to see corn again. Yet, producers have found ways to change and add corn to so many products that you cannot escape it if you eat any processed foods. The same goes for wheat, sugar, and potatoes.

Overfed on Sugar and Starches

Corn, wheat, sugar, and potatoes are the four big fall foods. They are normally in season or more available at the times of year when we gain the most weight. They can dominate your daily intake which is a huge problem since their nutrition content has dramatically changed over the past one hundred years. For example, the potato has much less nutrition because of the varieties selected for fast growth, high starch and sugar content, and method of preparation. This means there are fewer nutrients in the potato, less protein, less minerals, and less vitamins. This absent nutrient content and higher starch drives the insulin rollercoaster mentioned earlier.

The effect on your blood sugar is so profound that potato consumption by itself can contribute to weight gain and risk of diabetes. Increased potato intake can result in 1.28 pounds of additional weight gain for every increased daily serving. Potato chips cause the weight gain to increase to 1.69 pounds per serving in four years (Mozaffarian, 2011). When they are turned into French fries, the weight gain per four years doubles to 3.35 pounds for each daily serving. French fries are negative vegetables, meaning you have to eat one extra vegetable per day to make up for the impact of the fries.

What is a serving of French fries? That depends on whom you ask. Some consider the child's size as one serving, but many dieticians say ten skinny fries, or about 0.75 ounces (21 grams). Eating a daily serving sounds like a lot. The average child's size of French fries is 1.5 ounces (42 grams), or two servings. How about the large fries? That's about eight servings. Just one lunch or dinner with a large-size fries gets you to that one serving per day average. Two fast food meals per week are more than two servings per day. This works out to two pounds per year of weight gain from a couple of fast food meals with fries in a week, and this doesn't include what super-size fries or the rest of the meal including soft drink amounts to.

Remember, you are trying to find as many of your triggers for weight gain as possible. The impact from many triggers will add up over time. If this affects you, take note.

Instead of eating all fruits, most of us have our palates trained to recognize only apples, bananas, and oranges, and we eat these the most. They have become available all year long from places that never had the fruits growing naturally. Many are picked before peak ripeness on the tree or stored for a long time. Consider the tree as the fruits' mother and its connection by the stem as the umbilical cord, and you are eating a premature delivery. Yet, we have this as a regular practice in our fruits and vegetables.

Certain fruit characteristics are selected to make them more appealing and sell better. Size, color, and shape consistency are chosen over flavor and nutrition. Sweetness and sugar content is selected over what happens to your health when you eat it and what other nutrients are there. The perfect marketable fruit has been created without making sure the marketing hype is backed by real benefits.

Look at the fruits and vegetables in your grocery store. What are their harvest seasons? The majority are fall foods or picked well before their peak ripeness. This means the food never reaches its nutritional or flavor potential. Fall harvests are promoted as tastier because many fruits and vegetables are bitter in spring and summer. The bitterness has been thought of as bad but is due to the phytochemicals the plants produce to protect themselves from sun, pests, and other threats. Eating these give you similar protection. Have you been overwhelmed by mosquitos? When you were younger, they rarely bothered you. There is evidence this has to do with changes in diet (making you more appealing as a food source) and changes in their environment (eliminating some of their other natural food sources).

The Paleolithic Diet

Eating like our ancestors is suggested as how to be healthier and lose weight. In general, I agree with the concept of eating whole, unprocessed foods, but some people limit their palate or choices based on misconceptions about a Paleolithic diet. There is no one Paleolithic diet. Each region has foods specific to that region. Each season has specific foods. The idea there is one diet everyone used to eat to be healthy and lean is simply not true. Beyond this, the plants we eat today no longer resemble the versions of the plants seen in the past. Some of our common vegetables and fruits have undergone thousands of years of crossbreeding and selection resulting in what we have today.

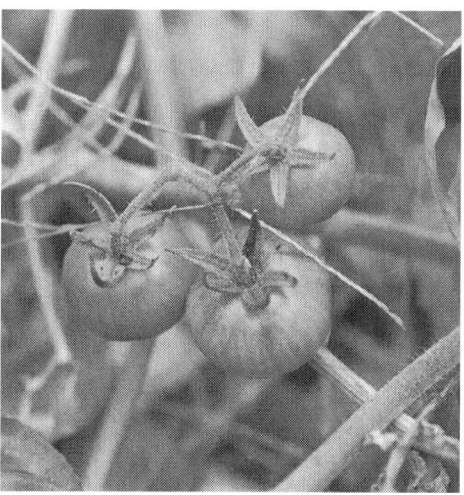

Wild tomatoes are more like berries than
the big fruit we know today.

We have seen a resurgence of more primitive forms of modern vegetables and fruits in recent years. Heirloom varieties are versions of plants we used to eat fifty to one hundred years ago. They retain some of the variation in size, color, flavor, and nutrients that used to exist in food but are still far from real Paleolithic forms. The basic premise of primitive eating is sound though. Reestablishing the balance of fats such as omega-3 and omega-6 as well as the balance of protein and natural unrefined carbohydrates is important. Consuming more variety like our ancestors and having that shift over the seasons is also a good goal.

If you think you are "eating Paleo", think again. If you are eating apples in Texas or bananas in Chicago, that's not Paleo. If you are eating wheat in Florida or oranges in Idaho, that's not Paleo. Foods have a time and place. If they are available at every time and every place, that's simply not Paleo and also not really as healthy as we think.

Nutrition and Agriculture

Even when we try to eat naturally we run into a significant limitation. Large-scale agriculture and production demands can deplete soil nutrition. Without replenishment of the soil over time, fewer minerals and other nutrients are there for plants to absorb and pass to us. For a long time, we focused on macronutrient content of food. How much carbohydrates, fats, and protein were thought to be the most important in nutrition. We next learned water and fiber were equally important and added them to the list of important nutrients. Vitamins and minerals are important to your health, yet the content of these micronutrients is frequently dismissed as less important to your weight.

A mineral such as magnesium is involved in over three hundred body processes yet is considered less important than the macronutrients, but it is crucial for good health. Like us, plants require these nutrients for survival and health. When they lack key nutrients, as happens with soil depletion and dependence on synthetic fertilizers, they don't pass the nutrients to us. They also can't make some substances, like phytonutrients, to protect themselves against infection or pests. Look up soil depletion online and you see a mix of opinions on whether this phenomenon is real or not. Supplement manufacturers fall on the side that soil depletion is real while agribusiness claims it's not. The idea of soil depletion makes sense and there is scientific proof to back the theory.

Scientific studies (Davis et al., 2004; Davis 2009) show a decline in at least six key nutrients (ascorbic acid, calcium, iron, phosphorus, protein, and riboflavin) from 1940s to 2000s in our produce. This is due to variety selection by farmers to get big, better-yielding, pretty fruits and vegetables while sacrificing flavor and nutrition. More importantly, the nutrition depletion is attributable to mineral depletion of soil (Davis, 2004). With the less flavor, processed food manufacturers use chemicals, colors, and flavors to replace the flavor lost along with these important nutrients. Traditional farmers and our ancestors knew crop rotation was important to allow soil recovery. Seasonal flooding and animal fertilizers also helped replenish the soil. Water flow is now extremely controlled and agricultural land is rarely flooded any more. Animals are generally kept out of the fields for fear of contamination of produce with bacteria. This means three key systems of soil replenishment have become less widely used.

How depleted is our soil and does it have an impact on our food? According to recent studies, the mineral content of agricultural soil has been reduced from four to ninety-six percent and organic carbon is as much as twenty-three to sixty-four percent lower in some places. Calcium alone is as much as ten to fifty-three percent lower (Rezapour, 2015). Imagine more plants planted in the same area and growing faster because of synthetic fertilizers. It's like having three people with straws sharing half a milkshake. How much can you suck out of that glass? It won't be too satisfying. Now imagine ten people trying to do the same thing. If each of them got a taste, they would be lucky. Plants crowded in a field to get the greatest yield are just like this example. Each plant sends down its roots in hope to get its fair share of the milkshake. Some people still believe plants are magically protected from this competition phenomenon.

When it comes to meat, this has been modified to resemble the fall version. Most cattle, chicken, and pigs are fed corn, wheat, and soy. These are not natural food sources for the animals and result in a higher percentage of fat, higher unhealthy fats, and a greater proportion of omega-6 as opposed to omega-3 fats (Rule, 2002). Animals eating natural forage, what they graze in the environment, have less fat and a greater proportion of healthy fat. The proportion changes by food availability, water, migration, and competition. Add to this that meat used to be extremely labor intensive. Tracking, chasing, dressing, and preparing an animal to eat took a lot of time and energy. The energy use has been eliminated. Further, the effort to catch the animal was quickly followed with an incredibly high nutrient dense meal. The organ meat was eaten first, often on the spot because it restored the energy and nutrition expended, and would spoil quickly.

Risk Factors for Weight Gain

Five risk factors for weight gain come from the food we take in (Urban, 2014). The problem is less with specific foods than how they are prepared and presented that makes the difference. Some risk factors seem obvious and others not so much. They are:

1. Consumption of liquid calories
2. Calorie density of foods
3. Variety of foods
4. Glycemic index
5. Percent of protein

Liquid calories are easy to consume and prepare. Soft drinks, coffee drinks, soups, shakes, and smoothies are examples of liquid calories. How quickly can you drink a large, highly sweetened coffee drink compared to a plate of healthy, natural food with the same number of calories? The problem is not recognizing its caloric influence into our diet. When you order coffee in the morning, you might get a muffin or bagel to go with it. You want a complete breakfast after all. Another big coffee follows the heavy lunch that made you sleepy in the afternoon. The calories continue to add up. Thirst is treated with soft drinks. You try to be healthy by making vegetable smoothies, and then add additional sweeteners or calorie dense items like peanut butter. You might purchase supplement shakes or meal replacements and end up taking them in addition to a full diet's worth of calories.

Calorie density is fitting more calories into a smaller volume. Butter is very calorie dense: little volume and high calories. Liquids are like this as well. Processed foods strip out the bulky components of foods such as fiber and water and leave them calorically denser than in natural foods. This is how the majority of these become transformed into fall foods. They are designed to pack as many calories on to your body as fat as quickly as possible, meaning you gain the same amount of fat with less food in less time.

Food variety is also a factor for weight gain. Variety can breed indecision and indecision leads to poor choices. The leading poor choice when dealing with variety of foods is "I'm going to try a little bit of everything." Inevitably, this leads to eating more than you would have. Think back to a party or holiday buffet. Remember the great foods with wonderful smells and color? You sampled a small amount of each, determined to eat within reason. A new pleasant experience greeted you when tasting each item. Then one food was amazing. You can't waste the food on our plate so you have to finish it but you want more of that one amazing food. Back for seconds and maybe thirds. Someone shows up with another dish and you can't be rude. Dessert is still coming. It's good, but did you try...?

This applies to processed and prepared foods as opposed to fresh or raw foods, but even "healthy" food can be less healthy through the wrong preparation. Weight gain from eating too many vegetables and fruits is still difficult. The difference with this risk factor of variety is a pound or two of extra weight gain. Even healthy food can result in as much as twenty-three percent more food and energy intake when too much variety is available at each meal (Stubbs, 2001). People trying to lose body fat eat less but can end up eliminating some of the healthy natural foods in favor of variety or processed diet replacements. Beware that this can feed into this same problem.

Glycemic index (GI) is how high a particular food raises your blood sugar. The number is compared to sugar or glucose which has an index of 100. Keeping to foods with a lower glycemic index helps stabilize blood glucose levels, preventing the peaks and dips that cause problems.

Blood Glucose over time

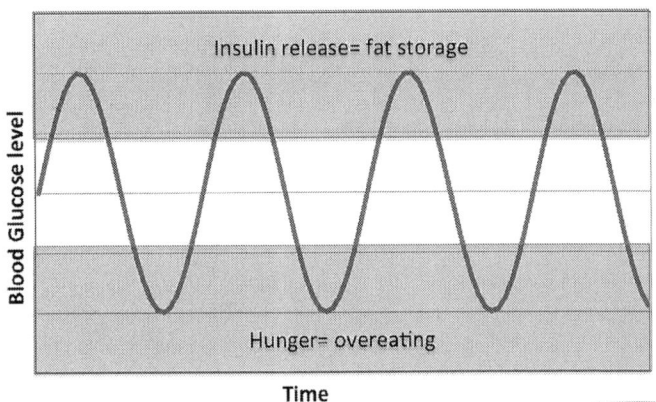

The highs cause insulin release and stimulate fat storage while the lows stimulate glucagon, epinephrine, and cortisol making you hungry. These numbers are important for people already overweight. People with normal weight or underweight and active are not as affected when it comes to weight gain due to GI. The GI is even more important if you are borderline or actually diabetic. While diabetics who eat low-glycemic foods may not achieve substantial fat loss, they do experience a reduction in glycated hemoglobin (A1C) levels indicating better control of blood sugar levels and a moderation of diabetic symptoms. This is without changing the total carbohydrate intake. All that has been done with eating low glycemic is adjusting how quickly sugar is released into the blood (Heilbronn, 2002).

Just for completeness, I want to include one new term that you may hear more about in the future. Because the glycemic index sometimes isn't precise enough to explain what actually happens in each person's body, a newer term—insulinemic index—describes the effect a food has on the insulin level in your body. A hormone like insulin (which increases fat storage) is obviously important to be aware of if you are a diabetic, borderline diabetic, or just concerned about weight loss. Making sure you know how you are impacting it with food is equally important.

I frequently hear how a person's cultural foods are unhealthy and they would have to give up their culture to eat low glycemic. The most common is, "I'm Mexican and our food is just unhealthy." I bet many Mexicans in Mexico would scratch their heads at this assertion by American-born or immigrant Mexicans. A 2003 study at the University of Baja California in Mexico demonstrated a low glycemic diet could be achieved using Mexican food and improve diabetes and health overall (Jimenez-Cruz, 2003). You do not have to give up your culture to eat healthy. Just make good choices and avoid the modern modifications made to food.

Remember glycation? Every time you allow your blood sugar to rise with high glycemic foods you create advanced glycation end-products (AGEs) that cause damage to your cells and lead to faster aging. Certain foods drive blood sugar higher—the high glycemic foods. The white foods, those with wheat and other refined starches, have a dramatic impact on blood sugar.

Protein Machinery

Your protein intake is extremely important for maintaining healthy weight. The entire metabolic machinery is mostly protein gears floating in water. If you don't have enough dietary protein, you can't use energy efficiently and store fat instead.

When you look at examples of some of these proteins on a microscopic level they look like the gears and levers of a machine or clock.

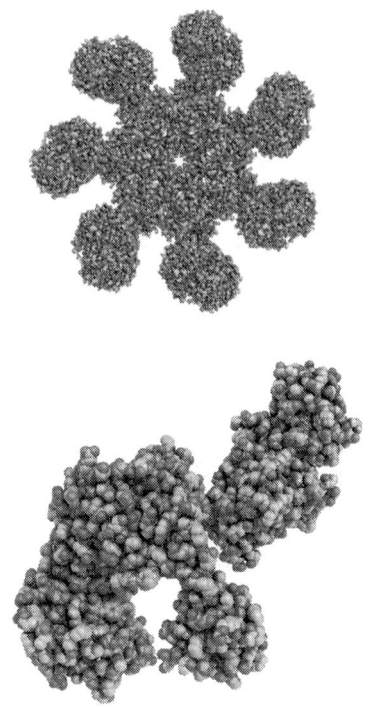

They are just like the gears and levers in a clock.

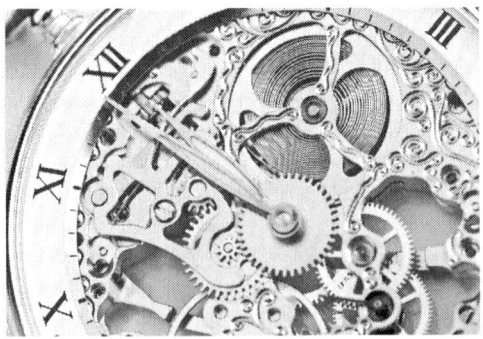

By not taking in enough protein, you can't produce all the parts of your fat-burning machine. By taking in too much of the substances that caused oxidation, glycation, or inflammation you rust, damage, or destroy some of the essential machine parts. It's important to eat enough protein to avoid losing gears from your fat-burning machine. A large portion of the population doesn't get enough protein and when they do it comes in an unhealthy package with excess fats or large quantities of carbohydrates.

So how do you get around these risk factors for weight gain?

1. Eliminate empty liquid calories to help avoid absorbing calories too quickly.
2. Decrease calorie density and increase nutrient density of your food by adding plenty of leafy vegetables, fresh fruits with fiber, and protein.
3. Decrease the variety of foods at each meal but increase the seasonal variety. Don't eat the same stuff all year long.
4. Reduce the glycemic index of the food you eat. Keep your blood sugar from peaking and crashing (see Resources for glycemic indices of food).
5. Increase protein intake to support muscle growth and a healthy heart, and to build your fat-burning machinery.

Let me be clear, I am not recommending low-carbohydrate anything. I also do not recommend flooding your body with too much protein. Low-glycemic means the sugars you eat should not increase your blood sugar and cause excessive insulin release. It doesn't mean cutting out carbohydrates. That is a recipe for disaster. For women, this will shut your fat burning down after five days, and for men, in addition, it kills testosterone production

You can minimize the impact of the fall diet. Free-range animals instead of corn-fed have a healthier fat content in the meat you consume for protein. This gives a greater opportunity for the fat to be used or eliminated. Reduce the four main fall foods—potatoes, corn, sugar, and wheat—and leave room for the vegetables and fruits that fight the bulge. Adding leafy vegetables with lots of fiber helps control sugar absorption. Increase the variety of meat. Beef, chicken, and pork provide very little variety, so add goat, mutton, turkey, dove, pheasant, deer, fish, buffalo, duck, goose, and shellfish to get a larger palate of protein. Variety is also important for vegetables and fruit. Eat the three fall fruits (apples, oranges, bananas) sparingly and replace them with alternatives in season. The fall fruits are the most commonly eaten in the U.S. and appear later in the year when temperatures get colder. While they have some health benefits, eating them all year long is not a good idea. Keep them in their season and add other fruits in theirs.

A Word of Warning

My student and friend, Myron, is a diabetic, but well on his way to losing his excess weight as he has identified many of his triggers and begun silencing his fat gene. He is excited to have clear goals and sees the possibility of doing some of the things he did when younger. Normally he has oatmeal for breakfast. Now his wife, having gone through our training, usually buys organic oatmeal but on one occasion, she couldn't find the organic and bought the plain, regular big brand oatmeal. Both were instant and unsweetened so the comparison was valid. They both were prepared the same way and topped with the same things but this is where the similarity ended. While the organic oatmeal raised his blood sugar to 160, the regular non-organic oatmeal caused a jump to 260, a one-hundred-point difference eating the same food, just organic versus non-organic! This isn't scientific, but illustrates there can be great differences in what we think is healthy. It also shows how someone can react to two different forms of the same food.

Is there evidence that this phenomenon in my friend is real and not just a fluke? Of course—I wouldn't have mentioned it if there wasn't. In a study out of Sweden, Granfeldt et al. (2000) examined the way that oats and barley were prepared. The conclusion was that more processing resulted in higher glycemic index of the cereal. If the oats were more steamed, roasted, or rolled thinner that may have caused this, but that doesn't exactly answer the question about organic versus regular crops causing differences in glycemic index. We already discussed the differences in nutrient content that can exist between organic and traditional grown foods. One of the minerals that is affected by both grain variety and method of planting is chromium (Su-Que, 2013). Chromium is well known to reduce the impact of sugars and starches on blood glucose and can help in glycemic control. The difference between organic and traditionally grown grains may be as much as ten-fold in chromium concentration! That has a huge impact on our blood sugar.

It's Not Fat, It's the Type of Fat

No fat, low fat, low saturated fat, and no trans fat are terms you have heard for the past few decades. We've gone through many wrong ideas and now the story about fat has started getting more interesting. Everyone agrees that not all fat is the same. There are definitely good and bad fats and the same sources can change in quality under different circumstances. You have probably read about trans fats in health bulletins as an example of unhealthy fats. Trans fats are byproducts of turning unsaturated fats such as vegetable oil into partially hydrogenated fats. This gives the fat a longer shelf life and a better melting point for use in food preparation. "Trans" refers to the orientation of a certain chemical bond in the fat. In nature, trans fats don't exist in great quantities. Instead, nature usually makes "cis" bonds.

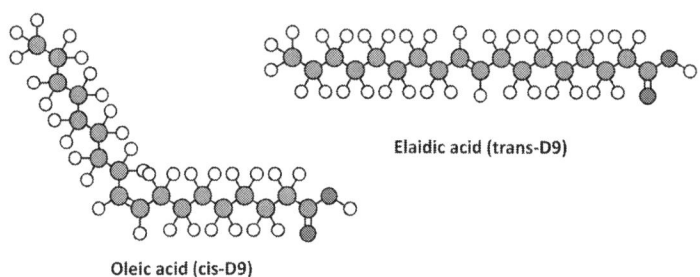

Elaidic acid (trans-D9)

Oleic acid (cis-D9)

These fat molecules have the same chemical composition but the orientation of the molecules in a bent shape makes a huge difference in how they function in your body. The cis form is needed for health while the trans form is dangerous to your health.

The U.S. government outlawed trans fats from foods after the world's oldest scientist sued the FDA in 2013, due to his research (Kummerow, 2009) proving their health risks. Dr. Fred Kummerow of Illinois, who turned 101 at this writing, has made huge contributions to science and health through his research linking trans fats to higher levels of low-density lipoprotein (LDL) or "bad" cholesterol. The LDL cholesterol has been linked to higher risk of cardiac disease. Trans fats should be avoided. As for cholesterol, it is extremely important in your body and the right type is actually critical for weight loss and good health.

As you eat trans fats, they are incorporated into your body cells at increasing levels. Trans fats in the cells prevent a process called esterification, which lets the cholesterol you eat be absorbed easier by your cells. If the cholesterol doesn't move to where it is needed in the cells, it sticks to where it's not needed when damaged by other food components (such as excessive sugar, which we'll get to later). That means plaque in your blood vessels and heart disease.

Omega-3 and Omega-6

Many other issues need to be considered. Humans evolved to eat animal fat and unprocessed plant matter and minimally-processed plant fats. Animal fat is not static. Animals gain weight and lose it over the course of the year. Fat formation is based on what is available for the animal to eat from season to season. This synchronization of weight gain and fat type reflect what is happening in the environment. The seasons tell your body to gain or lose weight. When fats have more of omega-3 from green leaves, this means spring and the time to lose weight. When you have more seed fats that are omega-6, your body senses it is fall and time to gain weight. More importantly, this determines what characteristics you express to deal with environmental pressures. The modern world has shifted the type of fats in your diet. This includes cooking fats, those used in processed food, and the naturally occurring fat on animals raised for meat.

We have moved from easily obtained plant fats and saturated animal fat from healthy animals to what we were never meant to eat. Fats are no longer synchronized to the seasons. Not only are most present day animal fats less healthy, we've been told to consume less. Instead, many people consume highly refined and processed vegetable oils and synthetically saturated fats such as hydrogenated oils. How many times have you eaten corn and thought, "Wow, this is pretty oily"? How about soybeans? Yet, we extract large quantities of oil from plants that have very little in a normally eaten serving. To do this there are harsh chemical treatments and high heat often changing more of the fat to trans versions!

Grain-fed cattle have less omega-3 fats than wild or pasture-fed cattle. Changing to grain reduces the omega-3 levels in meat by greater than seventy percent (Daley, 2010; Van Elswyk, 2014). Similar changes happen to eggs when chickens are grain fed. For most people, the changes are undetectable. For others, they experience better flavor with free-range meat that has higher omega-3 content. Being deprived of this source of omega-3, you need to make sure that you compensate in your diet. The rest of your diet has also been stripped of omega-3. Being aware of this and to reverse it is extremely important. In study after study, farm-raised animals are found to be at risk of having lower omega-3 depending on how they are fed (Rule, 2002).

If you visit a farm where the chickens wander around you may notice they eat anything that moves and will fit in their beaks. They are not limited to grains. The term "vegetarian raised" is stated as a positive for chickens, but that may not be an entirely accurate assessment. Free-range chickens not only eat grass and seeds, they also eat bugs. These are a rich source of protein and healthy fats. Chickens that eat bugs help reduce pesticide use around a farm and have higher quality meat with lower cholesterol and higher healthy fat (Sun, 2012). A natural diet is important for the animals you eat as well as you.

The types of fat determine what happens in your body. Healthier meats from animals with more natural diets will improve the healthy fats in your body. Practicing this regimen for as little as four weeks will change the fats in your body (McAfee, 2011). That's why it is so easy for unhealthy behavior to affect your health. On the other hand, you can have a positive impact by making good choices and sticking with them.

Why are omega-3s so important to good health? We hear frequently they improve immune function, reduce the risk of diabetes and obesity, improve mood, decrease depression, and improve learning and brain development, but how could one nutrient do so many things? The answer is actually pretty simple. Fats make up the majority of cell membranes. These membranes are the outside skin of the cell and hold it together. Without healthy cell membranes, everything going in and out of the cell is affected. If the membrane is not healthy, things don't move how they should.

Healthy fats also make the membranes more resilient, and allow cell surface receptors, which are made of protein, to detect the environment better and respond appropriately. These cell surface receptors are like antennas that detect signals from the environment allowing the cell to react appropriately or activate the right part of the DNA to adapt. The fats determine the shape and behavior of these receptors on the cell surfaces changing their ability to function or detect the environment. An example of a cell surface receptor is the insulin receptor that can be damaged or changed in configuration by the fats around and exposure to other damaging substances we eat resulting in diabetes.

Changing the types of fat in the membrane changes how the cells function. This difference determines what type of animals we resemble metabolically. As a group, mammals have a high metabolism that eats up extra calories to maintain body temperature, and makes them more active and able to tolerate wide ranges of environments. As a mammal, you benefit from this high calorie usage as well. The membranes of mammalian cells have a higher omega-3 unsaturated fatty acid composition than many other organisms. Reptiles have a slower metabolism and comparatively less polyunsaturated fats in their cell membranes and more omega-6 fats (Mitchell, 2007). By eating a certain way and being exposed to certain types of fat, you can transform into being more reptilian. The question is, which would you rather resemble, a reptile or mammal? Which is the better look? Kind of hard to accessorize with scales.

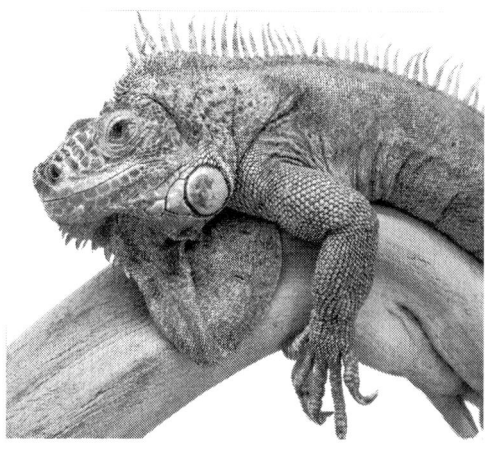

Making slight alterations in the fat molecule dramatically changes how it acts. For example, phosphatidylcholine is one of the fats found in cell membranes. Changing the position of one carbon atom alters the melting point from one hundred and thirty-one degrees down to five degrees F (fifty-five degrees to fifteen degrees C). This causes a fat to go from solid in a mammal to being liquid at normal body temperature. One of the most significant alterations is that substitution of omega-3 with omega-6 fats in your diet. Like I mentioned, this makes you more reptile-like. People have started having slower metabolisms like the reptiles their membrane fats resemble as a survival mechanism. A side effect of this transformation can be waxy, scaly skin some people suffer from. Not everyone is affected to the same degree. Some are severely omega-3 deficient and others are only slightly deficient.

Omega-3 fat deficiency is linked to obesity and continued weight gain. With low omega-3, there is disruption of cell membrane homeostasis (Bazan, 2011), the ability to keep the internal cell environment steady. Think of this as your cell's air conditioning and utilities. When the utilities get shut off what happens in your castle? Less work gets done and the ability to regulate cell function starts to fail. The membrane is involved in the detection of seasonal changes by cells and control of movement of materials in and out of the cell. When the membrane is unhealthy, this breaks down. Considering that the membrane is the means of communication between one cell and the next and how the cell detects toxins and defends against them, this is extremely dangerous.

Omega-3 fats have other benefits as well. The brain is composed of approximately sixty percent fat, so we are all "fat heads." A large portion of the membranes of brain and nerve cells are omega-3 fats. The amount of omega-3 fats and unhealthy fats in the membranes are extremely responsive to dietary changes so you are what you eat soon after you eat it (Orton, 2008; Sgoutas, 1970). Healthy omega-3 fats also compose part of the insulation of your brain wiring—the myelin sheaths around the brain cells. This is critical for the movement of signals in the brain. When the wire on your lamp loses its insulation, the lamp may short out. In the brain, shorts are manifested as changes in behavior, memory, and mood. If you don't get enough omega-3, you can't build or repair your wiring efficiently.

Deficiency of omega-3 fats is extremely common. We used to have omega-3 to omega-6 ratios of one to one in Paleolithic times, that's why I mentioned the Paleolithic diet before. This changed in modern times to a ratio of one to sixteen, one to twenty, or even as high as one to forty in some people. This affects healing, inflammation, and brain function. Any injury is harder to repair, and what we learn is harder to retain. Memory, mood, and behavioral problems are on the rise, along with attention deficit disorder

(ADD), attention deficit hyperactivity disorder (ADHD), autism, and depression. One of the most compelling reasons for this happening, is that fat and nutrition deficiencies are to blame (Antalis et al., 2006). Other factors, including genetics, play a role but don't explain the rapid rise and pervasiveness of these problems. While omega-3 is not a magic bullet, it is a good part of the solution and an easy place to start.

Omega-3 has an impact on brain development during pregnancy and can play a significant role in reducing injury severity and improving recovery from head trauma (Lewis et al., 2013). For this reason, the military has started supplementing soldiers to reduce the chances of traumatic brain injury (TBI). Omega-3 also has a positive impact on mood and its lack may explain the increases in depression in the population as a whole and particularly in soldiers and people who are overweight. Obesity, brain function, and mood are important, but they are not the only benefits of omega-3. It reduces the risk of premature birth by twenty-six to fifty-two percent. For women, if you want to be fit, lose fat, feel better, and have healthy pregnancies, you need this fat. Not all fats are bad and some are essential.

Omega-3 fats have several additional health benefits. Strong evidence (Fabian et al., 2015) shows that cancer, rheumatoid arthritis, and other conditions can be helped by the proper omega-3 to omega-6 ratio. This is because omega-3 isn't just in the brain, it's in every cell in your body. Liver tissue and the lining of your colon are sensitive to dietary changes because the cells are rapidly renewed and the tissues rely on fat for energy. Low omega-3 may be one explanation for the rise in fatty liver and nonalcoholic fatty liver disease, and irritable bowel symptoms.

That's not all. Omega-3 fats are involved in the body's ability to regulate inflammation. Omega-6 fats increase inflammation in the body and omega-3 reduces inflammation by decreasing the effect of omega-6. Muscle soreness, joint pains, fatigue, and poor recovery are partially attributed to the types of fat in your diet. Make sure you have enough omega-3 to replenish what you lack and turn off some of these chronic complaints. A weightlifter carries a large muscle mass on his knees and can still walk without significant pain. Yet, people carrying around excess body weight often complain of knee pain and difficulty walking. The difference is in the nutrition. The mechanical stress placed on the knees by lifting weights is greater than the slow increase in body weight. By changing the type of fats, you may decrease some of the inflammatory processes and pains you experience.

Replenishing omega-3 fats through diet or supplements can reduce the risk of obesity and help with weight loss (Bjursell, 2014). When preparing to lose body fat, replace your body's stores of essential nutrients (including these fats) as you cut calorie intake and exercise. Here's how to increase omega-3 in your diet:

1. Eat free-range beef
2. Eat free-range chicken
3. Eat free-range eggs
4. Eat free-range and wild game
5. Eat wild-caught deep-sea fish and sardines
6. Eat nuts and seeds
7. Eat organic, sustainably grown green leafy vegetables
8. Take a high quality supplement

Coconut Oil

Reduction in your healthy fats is a byproduct of the overall reduction of fat intake recommended through the last three to four decades. Excessive fat was an easy target for those trying to lose fat, but this is actually the wrong approach. Obesity and heart disease increased after the low fat dietary recommendations of the McGovern Committee in the 1960s and 1970s. Changing everyone's perception of what was good had an impact on health. The recommendations underestimated the importance of fat in your diet and only looked at the risks. Not only does fat have important roles in the body, but several things happen when you try to eliminate it.

This has been known for over eighty years but was originally received with much skepticism. Unfortunately, the same skepticism about the importance of fat has stuck with us until today. A diet without fat, particularly the essential fatty acids, causes all kinds of diseases and leads to a premature death.

With fat elimination, refined carbohydrates and artificial flavors are substituted to add back the flavor lost from foods. These may be more significant for weight gain than fat has ever been. Also, when fat is eliminated you lose a significant trigger for satiety. You eat and eat and never feel full. Ever see someone eat a bag of chips or box of cookies? Low fat? Ever see someone eat an entire stick of butter or drink a bottle of olive oil? Not likely. When you pair the fat with carbohydrates they are easier to take. Substituting fat with carbohydrates has a huge draw back. The high carbohydrate options are easy to eat and not very filling. They also contain flavoring substances that give your brain rewards, such as sugar, and make you overeat.

Since we were told saturated fat was bad for us, not only was saturated animal fat eliminated from most people's diets, but so was saturated plant fats. That meant coconut oil that is high in saturated plant fat was considered unhealthy. This couldn't be further from the truth. When it comes to weight loss, coconut oil is better than olive oil (St-Onge, 2008). Coconut oil is a great source for medium chain triglycerides (MCTs). The weight loss difference between olive and coconut oil is greater than four pounds over a sixteen-week weight loss program. Not only do the MCTs from coconut oil help with weight loss but they can reduce insulin resistance, decrease body fat, and reduce waistline and cholesterol concentration (Assunção, 2009; Kasai, 2003). Research (Sharma et al., 2014) shows that it may help with brain health, reducing the risk of dementia and Alzheimer's as well.

How can coconut oil do this? Recommendations of taking two to three tablespoons daily help with weight loss. At one hundred and seventeen calories per tablespoon, this seems impossible. How can you take in two to three hundred extra calories per day and lose body fat, reduce your waistline, and improve your cholesterol? This is what I mean by hidden reasons for weight gain and shutting off your fat genes. There are secrets built into your body chemistry you can take advantage of. With coconut oil, more is not always better. While I recommend taking two to three tablespoons per day, using more or less will not give the same results. Keep a food journal to document the amount and the results you get.

Let's look at how this unique fat can help reduce your waistline. Activation of your hunger hormones is determined by changes in what you eat. Coconut oil can modify the function of the hormones (Nishi, 2005). Less hunger hormones means less hunger and less eating. Regular long chain unsaturated fats (the "healthy" liquid plant oils you are accustomed to using) can inhibit or block the binding of thyroid hormone to its receptor (Inoue, 1989), but the MCTs from coconut oil don't do this.

The hormone is a key and the receptor is the keyhole. Blocking the receptor is like putting chewing gum in the keyhole. No matter how many copies of the key you have, you can't get the key in the hole to unlock it. This same problem with insulin receptors leads to insulin resistance and then to diabetes. Since the thyroid hormone is the master hormone that helps increase your metabolism, anything that blocks it from binding to its receptor will trigger weight gain just like in hypothyroidism. Using coconut oil helps keep the thyroid active.

Specifically, the main hunger hormone, ghrelin, has chemical modifications of the amino acids by coconut oil leading to inactivation.

Compared to olive oil, coconut oil gives greater weight loss and loss of upper body fat over a four-week program. This amounted to a three to four kilocalorie per minute (Kcal/min) difference in energy usage between the coconut and olive oil groups. Do the math to figure out what this turns into for weight loss. That measly three Kcal/min becomes 120,960 Kcal of extra energy usage over the four weeks, or over 34.5 pounds of weight loss. Hold your horses, cowgirl (or cowboy)! The real numbers for weight loss found in the study were much less, but the potential is there. The combination of MCTs and chili can boost the benefit for weight loss by increasing thermogenesis (heat production by the body) by as much as fifty percent (Clegg, 2013). Thai food with coconut oil and hot chilies may be just what the doctor ordered. Coconut oil also boosts immunity and its components can act as antimicrobials against some common bad bugs in your mouth and guts.

Coconut oil is considered a "super food." Be slightly skeptical when you hear "super food" as it usually refers to things people never ate before or in large quantities. I believe in moderation and look for benefits in commonly available items that give proven results. Now you know taking fat isn't the problem, it's the kind of fats that determine what happens in your body. But this isn't the end of the story.

The Need for Cholesterol

Along with fat is cholesterol. When you hear talk about one, the other is always close behind. Cholesterol has been maligned as the source of disease for nearly fifty years. You get cholesterol from the food you eat, but what happens when you don't eat enough? Your body is capable of making cholesterol in the liver. You can also reabsorb cholesterol from your intestine, more efficiently in the last part of your small intestine, when needed. When we think of cholesterol, we usually think of cholesterol level that's too high and the medications needed to lower it. Why do we have these ways of keeping our cholesterol high and why does it go up in the first place?

It's hard to lower cholesterol levels by limiting your intake or medications. The body has three separate mechanisms to increase cholesterol:

1. Dietary intake
2. Manufacturing cholesterol in the liver
3. Reabsorption from the intestine

Think about this for a second, when someone goes skydiving and they jump from a plane, how many parachutes do they have? They always have two because if the primary doesn't open you want a backup. Why? Because the consequence if a single parachute doesn't open is death. Whenever the risk is great of not having something work properly, you usually have backups. In your body, when you have more than one way to make, get, or keep a substance, it must be important. Cholesterol is another major component of your cell membranes. The cell membranes are only two molecules thick and fragile as a soap bubble. Your cells are susceptible to popping because of the fragility. By having cholesterol in the membrane, it becomes more flexible and less likely to pop. Without cholesterol, the membranes would require some form of protection like a stiff cell wall. Such a strong cell wall would turn you from animal to plant or fungus. You couldn't even be an animal without cholesterol. You'd be a vegetable, like carrots and celery.

Cholesterol also plays a role in nerve and brain development. In nerve cells, cholesterol is a key component of the myelin insulation around nerve cells. These communicate by electrical impulses, and the signals would quickly be lost without the proper insulation around your wiring. What happens to any electrical device when the insulation or the wiring breaks down? You start losing electricity and the device stops working. The myelin allows signals to travel longer distances along your nerves. It allows the transmission of signals down long pathways such as your spinal cord. Cholesterol is necessary to be any vertebrate, an animal with a spine, without this you would be a spineless carrot.

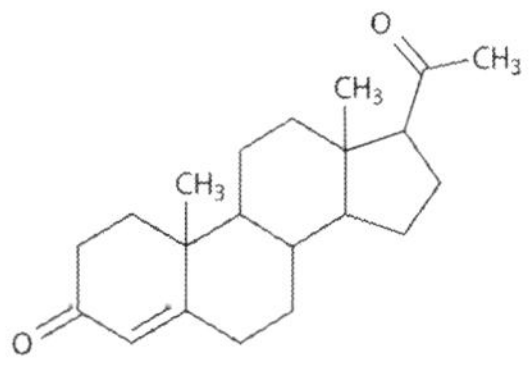

Progesterone

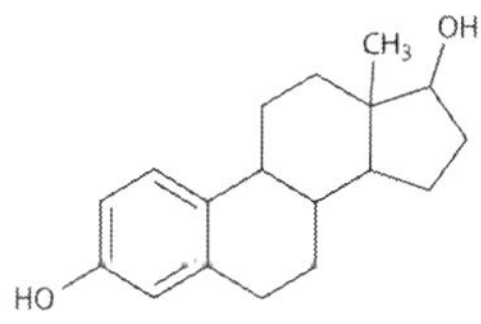

Estradiol

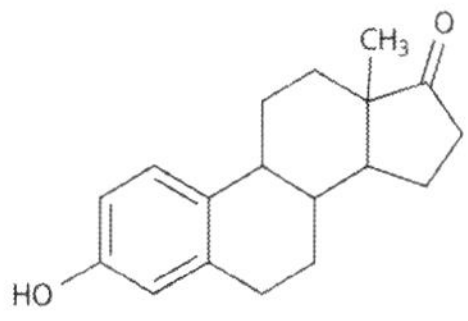

Estrone

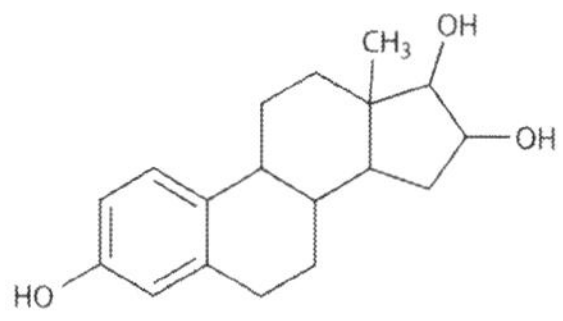

Theelol

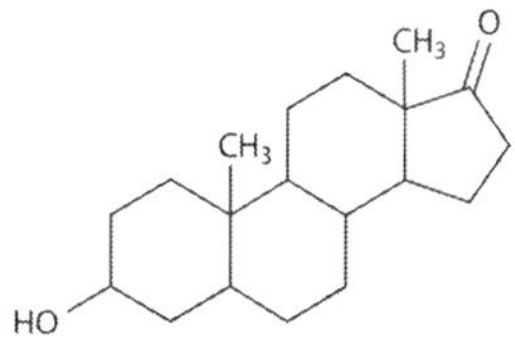

Androsterone

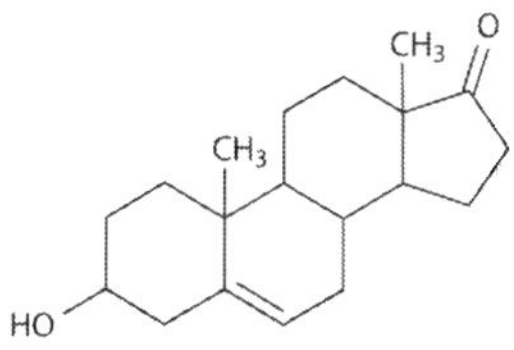

Dehydroepiandrosterone

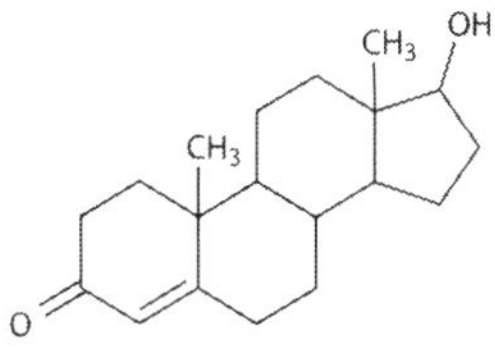

Testosterone

Cholesterol is one of the building blocks of many hormones. Without it, hormones such as aldosterone, cortisol, testosterone, and estradiol would be impossible to make. Your ability to handle salt with aldosterone would disappear, along with the ability to handle sugar and stress, and sexual development and function. Cholesterol is necessary for other important reasons.

Vitamin D, the sunshine vitamin, is made from cholesterol, and one of the most important vitamins in your body. Cholesterol has been maligned as a risk to our health, but you will find benefits the closer you look. Don't discount substances in your body and diet that are a natural part of food and nutrition because of misconceptions, what you are told, or because you don't understand their importance.

Cholesterol-lowering medications, the statins, function as heart protection only in a very small group of people. They work by blocking the liver's ability to produce cholesterol. Statins have a large number of side effects and complications. They reduce the risk of related deaths in younger men with a history of heart disease. Statins don't work as well for women or the elderly and don't prevent cardiac disease in healthy people with isolated elevated cholesterol levels (Vrecer, 2003). Their function isn't simply lowering cholesterol levels because they don't do that very well. Besides, lowering cholesterol levels doesn't protect against cardiac disease so the statins work through another method (Lim, 2014). They change the formation of the plaques that clog arteries so they become less thick (Banach, 2015).

Cholesterol is too important for many different body functions to be the real problem, and statins don't help all people. So why does cholesterol put you at risk and what is the difference between "good" and "bad" cholesterol? How do you improve the benefits?

LDL cholesterol is considered "bad" cholesterol, while HDL cholesterol is considered "good." Actually, there is no bad or good when it comes to cholesterol. Not having enough HDL increases the risk of heart disease, which is why it's considered "good." The "bad" is found in plaques that narrow arteries in atherosclerosis. This happens when the body is unable to process cholesterol properly or when it becomes damaged. The damage is usually caused by stress and leads to oxidation or oxidative damage. You may have heard this called "free radical damage." Some antioxidants reverse free radical damage or oxidation, reversing or preventing the process and improving the risks from damaged cholesterol. This seems to be one of the action mechanisms of statins, but remember it has many side effects. To reverse the damage to cholesterol, get the right combination of foods and supplements to achieve the same effect without the risks of statins. That means having enough anti-oxidants in your diet to keep the cholesterol from being damaged in the first place or taking adequate vitamin supplementation.

Maintaining Health with Vitamin D

English poet John Donne wrote, "No man is an island," but what does that mean? We are dependent on each other for many things in our lives. No one is truly self-sufficient, and some of the interactions in your body make you who you are and give you health or illness. No cell in your body is an island and all depend on each other.

Life started, or was created, in the simplest form of one cell and then multi-celled organisms. Your body is composed of approximately 37 trillion cells. Living things such as cells come together for a reason. There is a survival advantage to them working together. Similar to a village each of your body's cells plays a role to help the community survive and keep out foreign invaders.

Just like a village, there can be occasional conflicts. An individual from outside the village is recognized as an enemy invader and restrained, kicked out, or killed. A person may yell for help when a stranger is recognized and soldiers will show up. The signaling in the body is like this. When conflict happens, occasionally there are victims and innocent bystanders, which happens in the body as well. When you have an abscess or boil the dead tissue and pus are casualties of war. Some are warriors (immune cells) and others innocent bystanders. The analogy to a village doesn't stop there.

Sometimes, our soldiers turn on our own cells! Why do we get diseases where the body attacks itself? Villagers only fight each other when there are limited resources, like not enough money, food, water, mates, or homes. Imagine a scenario where this might happen in the body. When there is a scarcity in certain nutrients, water, or minerals, how does the body decide which cells get the limited resource? Certain things have to be distributed unevenly because needs are different. Some cells, like those making bone, demand more calcium. Nerve cells must have more omega-3 fats and cholesterol. When your cells don't get a share of the resources, they might rebel or go on strike. Body cells may start working improperly or stop their normal function. Renal failure, cardiac arrhythmias or irregular heartbeats, and psychiatric illness or degenerative brain disease are caused by the fight over resources.

In a village, you often have a group of stronger individuals responsible for defending the village: the police and military, the warriors of the tribe. These are the strongest and best armed of your citizens. When resources get scarce, they worry about their own wellbeing first. They abandon their posts to seek their own interest, and the criminals come out. In the body, these criminal cells are working completely wrong and may be harmful to the body, namely cancer. When the resource situation gets bad enough, things take a macabre turn. Your police and military enter the fight to take what they can for themselves. The immune cells attack the rest of the body, taking what they need as other cells give up what resources they have to survive.

Essential functions shut down when cells don't have enough resources. The proteins your DNA codes for will stop being made. The DNA is translated into making proteins that are the machinery for life. Proteins are how cells protect themselves, communicate with each other, release energy, and help gather more nutrition. When cells don't have enough protein, the body's machinery stops being made and repaired. Digestion, movement, heart function, and fat use will shut down. Proteins come from your diet, so the lack of function sets up another vicious circle of not having enough, making less body machinery and having less ability to absorb more. Proteins are one of the essential nutrients you get from your diet.

Fat is another important constituent of your nutrition. It's not just about calories. Every cell membrane is made of fat. The cell membrane that contains the parts of the cell inside is made of fat.

Omega-3 fats, among others, compose this. Without enough, you can't repair old cells or make new ones. The village faces severe problems when resources are lacking, like cancer, autoimmune disease, premature aging, and chronic aches and pains. Perhaps anti-inflammatory medications and immune suppressing drugs are unnecessary. Imagine if the answer has been nutrient deficiencies.

An entire field of medicine has developed to consider this concept. Naturopathic and holistic practitioners look at the body as a whole. They learn the impact of nutrition on the body and how to treat conditions with appropriate nutrition. This is a dramatic change from traditional western medicine of diagnosing disease and treating with medication or surgery. Incorporating these concepts into general medical practice is a great way to maintain health and support recovery from multiple ailments.

Don't run out and stop your medications just yet. Ask your doctor about nutritional interventions that might be helpful for your particular ailments. If they are unfamiliar with nutrition to take, seek out someone with experience. You can't just eat your way to good health any more because food isn't grown or produced like it once was, or contain the same nutrients that support the healthy function of your body. None of us is perfect in food choices and daily living. Since you have choice, you can still choose unhealthy things out of convenience. You should choose wisely and you should consider supplements of protein, fat, vitamins, minerals, and other nutrients essential to your health and survival.

Having good nutrition, good supplements and maintaining them gives the body the resources needed to rebuild. Supporting rebuilding of your village's resources takes time and the emergency measure of a medicine may not be required permanently. With these measures, you support healing and recovery rather than only treating symptoms. How do you know when you have enough? Plenty of studies talk about the quantities of this or that nutrient that promote health or avoid disease. These can be found online or in other books.

The basic principle is to take enough to reach the upper limit of normal for things you can test for and take enough to spill over in the urine for those that you can see. Many people worry about just making expensive urine with nutrient supplements, but this is a good thing. You can't predict when you will need the nutrients, so you need to be replete at all times. Spillover into urine tells you the tank is full. Since you don't have a full or empty gauge and don't feel any different once you have adequate amounts of nutrition, you need to make sure you are getting enough. You need enough not to just prevent deficiencies, but to reach extraordinary health.

The Sunshine Vitamin

In general, I don't recommend taking isolated vitamins. Most vitamins require multiple cofactors that act to help absorption and function as enhancers to help in conversion of the vitamin to its active form and to allow it to be used properly in the body. Without the cofactors, you waste your time taking the vitamins. Combinations work best when the vitamin is found with its cofactors. This is why you hear about the benefits of certain vitamins one day and they do nothing the next. Taking a single vitamin in isolation will not give you the benefits. Having the right cofactors and form of these critical substances is essential to your health.

Vitamin D fits with the theme of spring and sunshine and natural health. You might have heard about vitamin D recently as a panacea. While this isn't true of any one nutrient, let's explore why it's such an impressive vitamin and how valuable it is to your health.

Deficiency of vitamin D is associated with weight gain, insulin resistance, and other ailments. Many people are deficient in light and most of vitamin D is produced in your skin from sunlight exposure. Since we spend less time outside, we depend more on dietary sources of vitamin D. There are many natural sources of vitamin D in food, but how many people eat them? When was the last time you thought, I am going to eat this because it will give me plenty of vitamin D? Some people drink milk as a vitamin D supplement, but don't know it takes up to six to eight glasses of milk to meet the recommended daily allowance (RDA). While some dairy intake is important, studies show that more than two glasses a day are associated with obesity. Most doctors and many nutritionists don't know what the RDA is or where to get the target number.

The RDA for vitamin D is detailed in the following table (Institute of Medicine, Food and Nutrition Board, 2010).

Recommended Dietary Allowances (RDAs) for Vitamin D				
Age	Male	Female	Pregnancy	Lactation
0 – 12 months	400 IU (10 mcg)	400 IU (10 mcg)		
1 – 13 years	600 IU (15 mcg)	600 IU (15 mcg)		
14 – 18 years	600 IU (15 mcg)	600 IU (15 mcg)	600 IU (15 mcg)	600 IU (15 mcg)
19 – 50 years	600 IU (15 mcg)	600 IU (15 mcg)	600 IU (15 mcg)	600 IU (15 mcg)
51 – 70 years	600 IU (15 mcg)	600 IU (15 mcg)		
> 70 years	800 IU (20 mcg)	800 IU (20 mcg)		

Measuring vitamin D came from recognizing the development of rickets was due to vitamin D deficiency. Rickets is a disease where bones are softer or malformed from lack of mineralization. Any calcium taken in is not absorbed and used efficiently. Vitamin D's role was originally thought to be for maintaining calcium levels. Rickets was described as early as the seventeenth century, and attributed to vitamin D deficiency by the nineteenth century. The United States began fortifying milk with vitamin D in the 1930s. Before then, rickets was relatively rare.

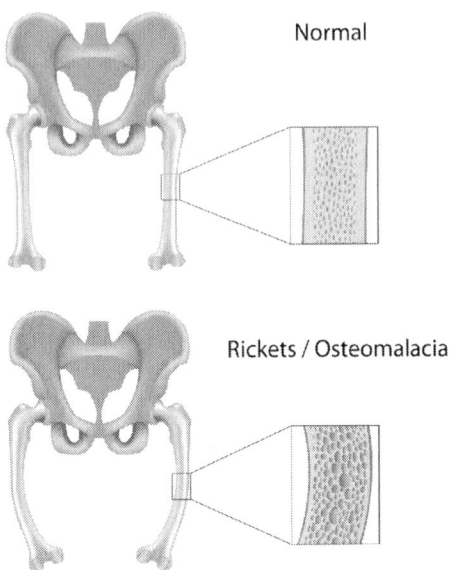

Normal

Rickets / Osteomalacia

What happened to prompt the nationwide drive for supplementing vitamin D? Rickets spread as city populations increased, diet was more limited, and exposure to sunlight decreased when people transitioned from a natural diet and outdoor living to city life and indoor living. Founded on the frontier and farming life, the U.S. shifted from the connection to nature to the creation of large expanses of paved, built, and shadowed areas.

For most people, rickets is a disease of a bygone era. Recent studies take notice of what people's vitamin D levels actually are and the impact these levels have on health. Many children and adults have critically low levels of vitamin D that increase the risk of rickets or are just above the level to prevent the disease. Overall deficiency has become common. I routinely check the vitamin D levels of my patients with obesity, as well as other conditions. In the last six years, I have seen one or two "normal" levels. "Normal" is the recommended level to prevent rickets, but not the levels to reduce the risk of other diseases associated with vitamin D deficiency.

If you have broken a bone recently or been without sun for an extended time, you should get your vitamin D level checked. If you complain of how pale you are after winter, get your level checked. If you are depressed, you can improve your mood with vitamin D. You must have adequate vitamin D when you are trying to have a baby or already pregnant. An athlete trying to heal, improve, or feel less sore after training or competing needs vitamin D, so get your level checked.

Rickets prevention requires very little vitamin D but this is not the only condition affected by the vitamin. Correcting vitamin D deficiency helps reverse or prevent conditions such as insulin resistance, obesity, and seasonal affective disorder (SAD). When you gain weight or try to lose weight, have abnormal sugars, or are depressed you should get your levels checked. Craving sweets and carbohydrates are other signs of low vitamin D. Having adequate levels of vitamin D during pregnancy has been shown to reverse or correct gestational diabetes. Diabetes during pregnancy can result in many complications for mother and child. Vitamin D has also been connected with decreased risk of colon cancer and breast cancer. Mood, cravings, weight gain, and cancer are some of the ways vitamin D affects you. There are quite a few benefits and yet, not only are most adults deficient, most children are as well.

Sources of Vitamin D

Vitamin D is easily supplemented by eating foods like line-caught fish and mushrooms, drinking milk or soymilk, taking a supplement and, most importantly, sun exposure. Trying to replace vitamin D using only one route is difficult and often doesn't work well when you use diet alone. You get real and durable results when you use a combination of methods of boosting vitamin D. However, there are many other vitamins and minerals your body craves and needs to be healthy that may be involved with weight gain and obesity.

Vitamin D in the diet comes from salmon, tuna, sardines, swordfish, cod liver oil, liver, eggs, and fortified foods. How often do you eat these? To prevent vitamin D deficiency, you would have to eat one of the big fish, such as salmon, every day and still take other sources. I love salmon but my appetite would disappear after eating it every day. As I mentioned, drinking milk for vitamin D requires six to ten glasses to meet your daily minimum requirement of six hundred to eight hundred IU (International Units). Milk is supposed to have one hundred IU per glass but can have as little as thirty-five to forty IU. That's over one thousand calories just from milk. Even though scientific evidence (Rozenberg et al., 2016) indicates that full fat, organic dairy is good for most people, I can't imagine anyone drinking that much. Cod liver oil supplements give you what you need but have you ever tasted or smelled it?

Another supplement many people rely on is orange juice with added vitamin D. A fat-soluble, oily vitamin is added to a sugary, water-based juice to make people think they are doing something healthy by drinking that juice. I'm not sure what trick of nature they're using to keep them together! This is not an ideal source since it relies on a sugary beverage with little nutritive value to get your vitamin D. Sounds like a marketing gimmick for juice manufacturers afraid of losing sales to a society leery of excess sugar than a real solution to a vitamin deficiency.

The biggest and best source of vitamin D is from sunlight on your skin. This source is free, natural, and all around us. Unfortunately, as outdoor time has decreased along with exposure to sunlight, your ability to make vitamin D has decreased as well. How do you know when you have enough vitamin D in a day from sunlight? Having arms, face, back and chest exposed long enough to gain a bit of color without burning is plenty. Obviously, the darker your skin color, the longer this might take. Don't think that having darker skin color prevents you from getting sunburned if you have been out of the sun for a long time. A friend with dark skin color, almost black, had been inside for more than a year except a few minutes at a time, and didn't realize until too late the mistake she had made. She suffered horrible sunburn after walking for an hour in the sun.

Build up your sun exposure over time, like working out. You wouldn't run a marathon the first day out or try to lift two hundred pounds without training your muscles. Yet, we expect our skin to be able to tolerate a visit to the beach without having been out in the sun twelve months prior when we were severely burned. We repeat this cycle and spend less time in the sun, and blame the sun for the increased risk of skin cancer when the lack of consistent exposure is the cause. In the marathon example, injuries or heart attacks are more likely due to the lack of training than the actual race. It takes time to prepare for anything, including sun exposure.

People coming from overseas to the U.S. underestimate the difference in outdoor time and the amount of sun they are getting. Many African immigrants and students often find themselves with unexplained ailments and depression. They arrive in places far north of where they used to live with much less intense sunlight. We often overestimate our time outdoors and underestimate its value, and can't recognize the symptoms of sunlight and vitamin D deficiency. In the U.S. there are few cities where people spend the majority of the day walking. Usually, it's a brisk walk down the street to the train, bus, or car to get to an indoor destination. Often we are covered from head to toe with little opportunity to soak up a few rays, even in summertime. Sun exposure is important to get daily.

The farther north you go, your skin makes less vitamin D. Above the thirty-seventh parallel latitude (horizontal lines on a map) you can't get enough ultraviolet radiation to make vitamin D. As leaves drop from the trees in fall, the ability to make vitamin D drops. Vitamin D production stops in winter in most places, and requires a combination of diet and supplements to maintain (Lips, 2014). The darker your skin the less vitamin D you make with the same exposure to sun. You normally store vitamin D in your fat, but if you are deficient, your stores can't get you through winter. However, your need for vitamin D doesn't diminish in winter.

Vitamin D uses the calcium in your diet to build bones and teeth, and supporting vitamin D levels requires calcium intake to spare vitamin D. They work hand in hand, vitamin D helping calcium and calcium helping vitamin D. Calcium absorption not only depends on vitamin D but also magnesium (Zofková, 1995). This makes supplementing exceedingly difficult and why, when studies are done on one vitamin alone, they rarely show benefits.

Obviously, there are challenges to get outside enough for the sun you need to make vitamin D without burning. Eating vitamin D is also a challenge, leaving you with supplements. Which form of vitamin D should you take? Vitamin D3 is the best to ensure you have the most active form. Since vitamin D is fat-soluble, taking it with fat makes absorption better. Vitamin K2 also helps the uptake and function of vitamin D, so formulas that include D3 and K2 are important (see Resources for recommended supplements). Adequate protein intake is also necessary for vitamin D. As I already mentioned most of us don't get adequate protein intake and those already with one deficiency are likely to be deficient in other nutrients. There are many requirements of vitamins, minerals, and other cofactors for proper absorption and use of any nutrient. If you miss any of these from your nutrition, vitamin D absorption and use may not be as good as it needs to be.

Vitamin Deficiency

Vitamin D can be hard to replenish with supplements. Some doctors give 50,000 or even 100,000 units of vitamin D daily to their deficient patients without seeing much benefit. The levels don't rise as quickly as they should with the high doses. A host of conditions occur in the body when vitamin D is deficient. Entire websites are devoted to revealing the benefits of vitamin D and the risks of not having enough (see Resources). Most recommendations for vitamin D are designed to prevent rickets but not focused on giving optimal levels to prevent other conditions. Vitamin D is critical in the repair of your DNA. Without enough, your machinery for fixing DNA damage doesn't work as well. In fact, the ability of the body to determine that a cell has damaged DNA diminishes and the risk of cancer and diseases such as diabetes and autoimmune diseases increases.

The websites devoted to exploring the role of vitamin D in your health, provide a large amount of data on its impact in reducing the risk of disease. There is a great misconception about the amount of vitamin D you require and how you should get it. Cancer risk, diabetes, and obesity are usually enough to convince most people that vitamin D is a good idea. Some of you may need more convincing. Vitamin D has been implicated in attention deficit hyperactivity disorder (ADHD) and autism. Inadequate amounts during pregnancy may increase risk of autism for the unborn child. A mother's vitamin D levels should be boosted before pregnancy to ensure the health of her infant. This is why we have seen a rise in autism, and it will continue in the U.S. and worldwide as habits and outdoors activities change. Africans rarely see autism in their countries of origin. Unfortunately, they gain the same risk of having an autistic child as American-raised individuals after living in the U.S. within a short period of time. They may recreate their traditional diets but the sun exposure is less and foods are not produced in the same fashion to retain nutrient content.

Vitamin D reduces autoimmunity and improves immunity against infection. It helps your body react more quickly to infection and has been shown to reduce the risk of influenza. That's quite a few benefits from one vitamin. You need enough. It's important to know what interferes with its production and absorption and that you have the right amount on a regular basis.

Inadequate cholesterol may interfere with vitamin D formation, but you not only get it from your diet, your body can make cholesterol. Cholesterol is not as bad as it has been made out to be and has many important roles in the body. When vitamin D levels drop with the change of seasons and decreased sunlight, the body tries to make more. To do this the body makes available more of the raw material for vitamin D, namely cholesterol. More cholesterol means a greater potential to make vitamin D. Are high cholesterol levels making more sense now? You must have heard someone complain about how high their cholesterol is despite cutting cholesterol from their diet, or going to the gym frequently, never mind being out in the sun. High cholesterol is the symptom of a different problem, namely vitamin D deficiency (Aranow, 2011).

We also know that correction of vitamin D levels can help improve insulin sensitivity in children and adults (Belenchia, et al., 2013). The benefits of this are simply great. Not only does it take you farther away from diabetes, but it also allows you to use your carbohydrates for fuel in the muscles instead of storage as fat on the body and liver. Since insulin sensitivity means lower overall insulin levels in response to foods it means less overall fat storage effects. Weight loss becomes slightly easier. Recurrent hunger is less and energy levels improve. You probably won't get "hangry" when you miss a meal or two.

Another interesting phenomenon with vitamin D is its important relationship with pain, muscle recovery, and perception of discomfort. Why do your muscles and joints ache in winter? Why is it harder to move around like you feel older? This may be a sign of low vitamin D levels. Patients recovering from surgery were studied and found to be more likely to have chronic pain with lower vitamin D levels (Matossian-Motley, 2016). Many studies confirm this association although the cause has yet to be firmly established. One study linked one hundred percent of patients showing pain with vitamin D deficiency. They even found the levels of vitamin D were not affected by season like normal. This is troubling to think there's no longer variation between the seasons when we should make lots of vitamin D and the seasons we don't. People have separated themselves from the seasonal cycle and this is proof (Plotnikoff, 2003).

We expect the people most passionate about promoting health and open to thinking of health in a holistic manner are less likely to have low vitamin D levels. Who am I talking about? Young physicians, the new students of science and health keen to change the world and have an impact on the lives of their patients. These individuals are interested in their own health as well. The reality is they fare no better than the rest of the population. One study demonstrated that between seventy-five and ninety percent of young doctors from diverse ethnic backgrounds were deficient in vitamin D (Manickam, 2012; Ramírez-Vick, 2015). How does this affect their decision-making process when dealing with your health? If they know the impact of vitamin D on health and are unable to maintain their levels, what risk do you have for low vitamin D levels?

Vitamin D is no panacea, despite its impressive benefits. It's one cog in a complex machine that is missing for many people. Having too much of a good thing doesn't mean you get healthier. Excess vitamin D is toxic and some diseases are increased with higher levels. Don't just gulp down any supplement without knowing how much you should have. Everyone requires a different dosage and the amount of body fat you have determines how much you are able to store. You need other vitamins and minerals, fats, proteins, and good carbohydrates as well as water to make the whole system work. Many substances necessary for your health and disease resistance have yet to be identified or carefully studied.

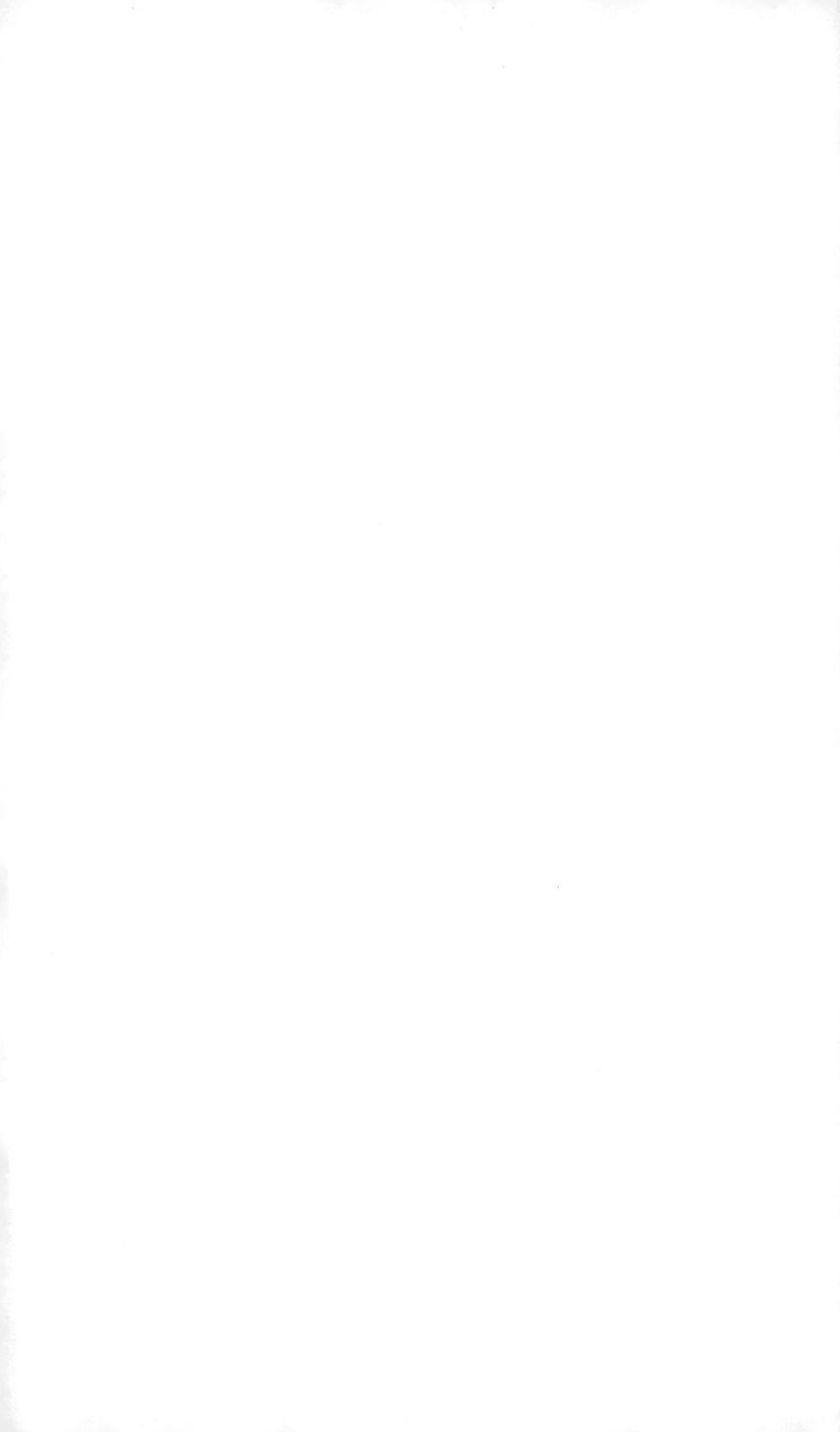

10

Drink Water, Not Sport Drinks

Drinking water is essential for maintaining a healthy weight and makes weight loss possible. It is the medium your body's cells use to carry nutrients, including vitamins and minerals, and distribute them appropriately. Just by drinking water, your resting energy expenditure can increase to result in more than two pounds per year of weight loss (Dubnov-Raz, 2011). Water has an impact on your blood flow and how you eliminate wastes from your urinary system and colon. The appearance of your skin is dependent on water intake. Chronic dehydration is a problem for many people. They underestimate their water needs and this results in inefficient metabolism and aging of the skin.

Water is always the best choice for drinking. Unfortunately, many people use nonnutritive beverages as their liquid sources and take most of these at meal times. This contributes to, and is associated with, higher calorie intake. Liquid caloric intake is one risk factor for obesity. Not drinking water, or drinking with meals, puts you at risk for being overweight. Drinking water has another great side effect. Children who drink water are smarter and have brains that function better (Benton, 2011). Setting the example for children is reason enough to drink water, but even 1-2% dehydration can result in worse brain function in adults (Riebl and Davy, 2013).

We have all been told to drink more water, usually six to eight glasses or one-half ounce per pound (30 mL per kg) of body weight for the average person. By adding this water, you get 4.4 pounds (two kg) of weight loss per year. It takes little effort and cost, and will continue as long as you do it. Five years of improving your water intake can be twenty-two pounds of weight loss you would otherwise struggle to achieve. This makes a huge long-term difference when added to other healthy activities. A friend of mine joked that drinking his water made him run to the bathroom more frequently, and gave him more steps and exercise over the day. Hey, we'll take that, too!

You may realize how much water you need when dealing with excess body weight. The amount is less for excess body fat. Figuring out your lean body mass and fat mass will help. A scale that tells you your body fat percentage can be purchased at your local gym or sports equipment store. Fat cells have less water than muscle cells and require less water. They still require water but not quite as much. Cut the calculated amount in half for the body fat percentage. For example, someone who weighs 300 pounds and has a body fat percentage of fifty percent would have a lean mass of 150 pounds and a fat mass of 150 pounds. The water for the lean muscle mass would be 75 ounces and for the fat mass would be 38 ounces for a total of 113 ounces. This is important because too much water can lead to water intoxication. It only takes six liters of water to kill the average 165-pound person. Too much is not a good idea but it's really hard to get there with the above calculation.

When you drink six to eight glasses of water a day, initially you might gain weight but then it drops rapidly. Stick to the recommended amounts and take a one or two-day holiday each week from the strict requirements. Studies indicate that when you hydrate like this your insulin receptors work better, meaning less insulin resistance and improvement of diabetes. Since insulin resistance and diabetes are risk factors for weight gain, correcting insulin receptor function helps speed up your weight loss. Water intake also increases energy use and improves fat loss (Henriksen, 2007; Mathai, 2008).

When people don't trust the water supply, don't like the taste of the water, or are unaccustomed to drinking water, they make other selections. Children follow adult examples and choose what's easily available and tastes good. Setting an example and making a healthy choice for yourself should be your goal. But the water has to be good for you to drink it. Many people won't drink water because of how it tastes in their local area. With all the bottled and purified water available, this isn't an excuse anymore—but what acts on the taste of water?

Water taste is affected by minerals, dissolved gases, and contaminants; by the types of pipes it travels through; or the containers used to store it. Flint, Michigan in the past few years had a huge water contamination problem that illustrates the point about distrusting your water source. This was due to contamination of the water and corrosion of the pipes that led to further contamination. Flavored drinks overpower these same taste contaminants. The flavor consistency between one bottle and the next makes artificial drinks very attractive for many people. Instead, we should find sources of clean water and store in containers that won't change the taste or contaminate it.

Most water is stored in plastic bottles. Aside from health risks of Bisphenol A (BPA) and other plastic residues leaching into the water, the flavor can also be changed. But that's not all that happens in plastic bottles. Within three to four days, the bacterial count from fresh spring water in a plastic bottle is the same as in the first part of your colon (Bischofberger, 1990; González, 1987). I don't know about you, but I certainly don't want to be drinking water with the same amount of bacteria as poo! Wonder why the water tastes funny? Maybe this explains it.

If the type of bacteria in your diet helps determine your weight, you also don't want random bacterial contamination from the water itself or a bottling facility in what you drink. You want natural, healthy food sources of good bacteria, and clean water. Purified water doesn't have the bacterial risk. Spring water from the source is usually good for you, just not after storing in plastic. Glass and stainless steel containers don't carry the risk of plastic residues or bacteria if they are kept clean. Nor do they change the flavor.

Ice and Iced Drinks

One modern factor that plays a role in energy and temperature regulation is our use of ice. We have cold drinks and foods available like never before. I have friends that have never had a drink without ice, other than coffee or hot chocolate. Everything has to be chilled to extremely cold temperatures. Does this have an impact? Everything you do will have an impact on how your body works.

Most of us have been taught cold drinks burn calories. We add ice to water and every other drink we can think of, including coffee and tea. Iced tea was the staple drink when I was younger and my family first moved to the south. It was unusual to me that anyone would ruin a good cup of tea with ice. Jump forward twenty years and we drank it on a regular basis in my family. We expend about twenty-five calories warming up a glass of ice-cold fluid when we drink it. Unfortunately, the extra heat generated from metabolism would have dissipated anyway to keep your body cool. There is no real benefit. Drinking a gallon of ice water doesn't work how you hoped it would. Don't worry: the water, not its temperature, increases your metabolism.

Many people drink ice water because of the refreshing sensation it gives. This shuts off your thirst center. You are satisfied and your thirst is quenched with less water. Even when you are hot and thirsty you drink less. Your mouth can't tell what you're drinking to quench your thirst. When placed over ice, any drink affects the thirst center. Sugary or dehydrating beverages such as soda over ice seem satisfying. See the hot and cold beverage experiment in the chapter, Temperature and Metabolism, for details. This illustrates how temperature affects your taste. A sugary beverage doesn't taste as sweet and seems to quench your thirst temporarily. Soon the thirst returns and if you continue drinking cold, sugary beverages, you get into a vicious loop of temporary thirst quenching with more sugar intake. That's why the giant ice-filled soda cups at the quick marts are so popular.

When is ice okay? When is cooling helpful for activity? The average person rarely needs additional help to stay cool to improve performance. By allowing the body to regulate its own temperature, you become more comfortable under those conditions. Elite athletes sometimes need an additional edge. Their goal is not to lose weight but rather to improve performance. Athletes that perform long distance or endurance type events in higher temperatures would benefit from a cooling drink or other method of body cooling (Wegmann, 2012). This is because seconds make a difference at that level. It is rare when a fraction of a second makes any difference for the person exercising for fitness or weight loss.

Ice also has a distinct side effect on stomach activity. Your stomach empties slower when you drink ice-cold fluids (Sun, 1988). Anything you eat will sit and mix longer, meaning greater absorption of the same food. It doesn't end here. The reason we like cold drinks is the sensation in our mouths is refreshing. Like I mentioned, cool water shuts off your thirst center and makes you drink less (Brunstrom, 1997). If you drink one glass and feel refreshed, you never have the second glass you need to quench your thirst and fully rehydrate. This dehydration makes you tolerate cold better. Good hydration makes you tolerate heat better.

Drinking isn't the only way to use water for helping with weight loss. Swimming or exercising in water also helps. Exercising in water allows heat loss to happen thirty times faster than in air. This is why you get cold fast when you get wet. Maintaining your temperature becomes a challenge even at higher water temperatures. Competitive swimmers need greater calorie intakes than the average athletes. Michael Phelps was known to down ten thousand calories or more a day and he wasn't doing more exercise than any other competitive athlete, he was just training in the water more. If you wonder whether a water aerobics course is worthwhile, the answer is yes.

Marketing Energy

Marketing drives the use of energy and sports drinks. While some may be useful for elite athletes, normal people rarely require their use. The salts and minerals necessary to maintain health and compensate for sweat losses come from food. In fact, one study links sports drinks with sugar to long-term risk of diabetes (Hu, 2010). Those who consume beverages with high sugar content when participating in fitness activities are likely to consume other unhealthy items in their diet. Energy drinks do very little to maintain natural energy levels and cover up fatigue, poor nutrition, and deconditioning at the root of the problem. They also temporarily cover hormonal deficiencies that cause low energy levels. The health risks of these drinks are not fully known. They have many components that may have toxicities that contribute to other health problems (Seifert, 2011).

Marketing of sugary beverages including sports drinks has been used to sell you many products that promote weight gain. Consider the list of bogus, lose-weight-quick solutions. The confusing messages leave you uncertain about what is truly healthy and what is not. Frequently, companies meet their goals of selling more by blurring the line between truth and fairy tale. They convince themselves they are doing the world good by providing consumers with "good taste," variety, and choice. Look carefully at the process of marketing. None of us are immune to the hype, but being an educated consumer will reduce the impact of these psychological tricks.

How Marketing Works

The mind plays a significant role in how your body functions. An intricate intertwining of thought and biology in the brain alters perception, thought, and future behavior through a complex system of reinforcement and gene modification. This can lead to overeating or the unbalanced eating that causes obesity.

A former soft drink manufacturing executive told me about the practices used by the company in marketing and sales. They spoke of market share, which is not surprising for a commercial enterprise, but also about "stomach share" as a measure of their success. The goal was how much of your stomach could they take over through their products. What marketing, methods, and new products could they use to get you to fill more of your stomach? The "super-size" scheme was a result of them wanting to move more products. It's scary to think these large companies are working to find the best way to get you to voluntarily displace nutritive food with a synthetic concoction of addictive and harmful ingredients. It almost sounds like drug dealing.

Manufacturers of fast and junk foods resist calls to reduce the negative impact of their products. They tout personal freedom and choice, and invoke individual responsibility and activity as the solutions to the excess they distribute. That's like the tobacco industry stating that lung cancer from their cigarettes isn't their fault, it's the smoker's fault for not coughing hard enough and taking vitamins. The similarity to tobacco doesn't stop there.

They use images of young people, fitness, refreshment, happiness, and attractiveness to sell what should be unsellable. This is how the tobacco industry once advertised their products and how they market vapor devices today. Convince people that what they sell will put them into a peer group of young, healthy, vibrant individuals and it becomes an attractive product. By labeling products with healthy-sounding information, it makes the foods being marketed sound better than they are. When you see "sugar-free," "fat-free," "good source of healthy fiber," "packed with vitamins and minerals," "good source of vitamins and minerals," "good source of whole grains," or "all natural ingredients" on a package, it's guaranteed to be hype. Nothing that is processed and put into a package retains the healthy benefits of the original ingredients. Processing through excessive heating and the addition of flavorings makes these foods dangerous.

Junk Food and Rewards

I've seen more children coming to the emergency room for Flamin' Hot Cheetos ingestion than any other source of abdominal pain. Your poor brain doesn't have a chance against modern chemistry. The combination of rapidly digested carbohydrates, salts, and spice trigger the dopamine and endorphin receptors in our brain. Despite the pain and discomfort you get from eating them, these foods reward your brain. No wonder your children get cranky when you take away sugar or snacks. Most children can't resist spicy, crunchy, salty snacks any more than adults. The problem is the responses aren't as great the next time so it takes more of the drug to get the same effect. Just like illegal drugs, these foods sabotage your reward system and make you take more to get the same effect.

A good friend opened the cabinet in our doctor's lounge where snacks are kept and exclaimed, "Oh, Cheetos. I know they are bad for you, but I just can't resist." This is music to a marketer's ears. The win for marketers and food scientists that created this concoction means a huge loss for you. For a mature individual who is a highly educated doctor to have his brain hijacked by a bag of orange-colored puffed starch is amazing. We are all at risk of becoming zombies like this: no control over our actions, simply driven by our brain chemistry to repeatedly eat the same unhealthy foods.

You are also being tricked by changes in food labeling. Portion sizes have grown over time, even for the same products. They began to rise in the 1970s and have continued to increase. This correlates with the rise of obesity (Young, 2002). Between the 1970s and 1990s, a third of the diet eaten outside the home increased to almost fifty percent. Portion sizes in some cases doubled or increased to eight times the original size (Young, 2007). Since weight gain is correlated to the number of servings of food items like potato chips and French fries, having serving sizes equivalent to multiple servings puts you at risk even when you think you are doing pretty good.

A standard child size of French fries is actually two servings and the larger sizes are much more. The package you are sold is intended for eating in a single sitting but contains anywhere from two to five servings. When given a palatable food that stimulates your brain reward system positively, stimulates your major fat storage hormone system, and then multiplies the servings, you gain weight. This seems innocuous but translates into as much as forty pounds over a ten-year period.

Today we are sold a new bill of goods described as "more realistic" and "less discriminatory" with the recent appearance of plus-sized models. While we have been submitted to decades of overly thin, airbrushed, and photoshopped models, the recent attempts to classify being overweight as normal are disturbing. No matter how beautiful people are, over weight is never healthy unless the person always eats healthy, takes supplements, exercises regularly, and has full mobility, and no limitations or signs of disease associated with the weight. This also means the distribution of fat in the thighs and legs as opposed to around the waist and chest.

Marketers tap into the psychological desire for people to fit in and be accepted but they are not doing it for the noble reasons of equality or human compassion. Discrimination based on weight is never acceptable, but the marketers are only finding another audience to sell to and not helping the situation. Showing plus-sized underwear models is exchanging one distorted view for the other extreme. There is a happy medium and a real health risk associated with too little or excess body fat. No matter how much you want to accept this "friendly" marketing ploy, remember it's just another cartoon tiger peddling sugarcoated death.

Some companies have caved in to public pressure and try to remake their images as healthy. Social responsibility and caring for people should come because it is the right thing to do. Eating healthy and choosing to use healthy ingredients in food should be done because it's right, not required. Imagine if companies had to charge the cost of the health problems they cause with their foods. The value of a one percent reduction of obesity is a saving in health costs of almost three billion dollars in Canada alone (Krueger, 2014). Add this to the cost of the foods that trigger weight gain and it would help reduce health expenditures. Right now, you pay for cheap, convenient fun food in your weight, health, and long-term expenses. In the U.S., this one percent obesity-reduction translates into a savings of at least forty-six billion dollars annually.

Do you want others controlling the way you think and eat or do you want to make choices that are healthy for you? This question cuts to the core of what the marketers are doing. They use psychological tricks at times of the day when people are most vulnerable to suggestion. If only they would use their powers for good. Instead, they promote addictive ingredients in more clever and ingenious ways to achieve higher sales and consumption. Marketing has become such a part of our society that we hardly question it anymore.

Solving the Problem at Home

The solution is to give up media. When you take away the influence of media, you have more free and productive time. Giving up excess TV hours creates time to learn and read, and to exercise and prepare healthier foods. You can spend more time with your spouse and children to talk, bond, and resolve problems. Just like fast food for your body, media degrades your brain by playing off the same pleasure centers that drive you to overeat. Ever find yourself surfing the net and looking at the Facebook posts from people you hardly know? Catch yourself playing that colorful video game that draws you multiple times per day? These are no different than chocolate or French fries. They taste good and make you feel good now, but waste a great opportunity and decrease your health overall.

Set the electronics down and turn off the TV. Like anything in your life, if you feel it's important you should schedule time for it. Having set hours to use the media is the first stage of controlling its use. It will also make you aware of the hours and minutes that tick away while you use them. While you can reclaim your health and lose excess body weight, time can never be regained. Was that movie or TV show worth the two hours of your life? Has it added a value or insight to improve your life, deal with others better, or improve your family life? Only the rare fast media program does any of this.

When you reach for a device, stop and count ten deep breaths. Ask yourself, *Is this the best thing for me to do right now or is there something more important, urgent, or better?* This simple one-minute trick will save you hours and create an abundance you didn't know existed. People often ask me how I fit so much in my day. This is my secret weapon. Just a short pause frees my mind and gives me back the stolen hours I miss at the end of the week. By actively deciding what is the best thing to do, I keep from wasting hours on distractions. That isn't to say I never watch a movie, TV, or use Facebook or play games. Instead, when you are more selective, you get more done in your life and enjoy recreation without guilt.

Marketing can hijack your brain and contribute to the activation of your fat genes. What are the solutions? How do we tap in to our brain reward systems and activate your weight loss DNA for better health? The following list makes the process easier and will lead you to greater levels of accomplishment.

1. Stop eating salty, processed snack foods. If it's not in your house, you can't eat it. Having them on a special occasion gives you additional brain rewards without making addictions or added weight gain.

2. Never eat while watching TV. You will be unconscious of what you eat and how you chew, and susceptible to suggestion of commercials.

3. Eliminate watching or listening to ads. The suggestions built into the marketing are subtle and sophisticated. It's hard to keep those messages out of your head.

4. Decrease TV-watching. This will give you more time for family, friends, work, self-improvement, and healthy food preparation. Not watching the food advertisements also help avoid

the psychological tricks that make you crave things you don't need or really want.

5. Let social success and societal contribution give your brain chemical rewards. You will continue to feel good about these actions and make others feel good.

6. When in doubt, pause and take a few deep breaths and think, *Is this the best thing to do right now or is there something more important, urgent, or better?* Add to that, *Should I be eating this or is there something better?* Choose good for your mouth and body, not just your mouth.

7. Ignore the claims of "healthy," "good source of...," "reduces heart risk," "reduces cholesterol," "low salt," "low-fat," and other marketing gimmicks. If it's processed, it's not worthwhile.

Being aware that marketers know what is going on in your head is important. It keeps them from being able to hotwire your brain and leaving you with a wreck after their joy ride. Well, it doesn't keep them from doing it but now they have to do it with your knowing complacency. You were an unwitting accomplice in ruining your health every time you watched the commercials and opened a bag or bottle of the easy snacks marketed as fun and hip. Now that you know, you can prevent becoming the patsy to the marketers.

Boosting Metabolism Through Exercise

As you can see there are already many factors from the environment and our food that contribute to weight gain and can be blocked or eliminated to help with weight loss. Your nutrition is absolutely critical. While it is difficult or nearly impossible to exercise your way to weight loss, exercise has a huge impact on how energy is used or stored in the body. Exercise training can boost the metabolism by nine to eleven percent or more (Lemmer, 2001; Jabbour, 2015). Conversely, deconditioning and lack of activity makes an active metabolism slow down by the same amount. A person with a sedentary lifestyle who's supposed to eat a 2000-calorie diet burns about 220 calories less per day to meet his or her predicted needs. This translates to 80,300 calories per year or twenty-two pounds (10 kg) of added weight per year. You see how quickly it adds up? Only thirty minutes of intense activity is necessary to lose those calories but five minutes to eat them.

Two hundred and twenty calories is equal to one donut or a quarter cup of peanut M&Ms. If you ate either one every day you would not be surprised if you gained weight. What else equals 220 calories?

- Thirteen servings (6-½ cups) of green beans
- Twelve servings (six cups) of kale

- Five tomatoes
- Twenty-two servings (eleven cups) of broccoli
- Two bananas
- Two apples
- Six servings (three cups) of pineapple, raspberries, or strawberries

Each has about 220 calories. You could eat a lot of food for the same amount of calories. When you choose to be inactive, you are deciding not to eat more food and be satisfied. A limited intake also limits the nutrition you get from the food and not just the calories. Unhealthy choices have a greater impact than just the calories. They also strip you of the opportunity to take in the nutrition that helps prevent weight gain.

Unhealthy eating means either overeating unhealthy foods or eating a lower volume of food than you would otherwise, and getting less nutrition. It has very little to do with calorie intake and you have more cravings. You will always feel hungry faster than when eating healthy. By including more nutrition in the foods you eat, you feel fuller, have fewer cravings, and feel better overall. You can also afford to eat some of the "cheat" foods without any problem, but you probably won't want to as much. While eating healthy accounts for eighty to eighty-five percent of weight loss, you also want to take advantage of the output through activity.

We have heard how we have all become lazier and less active than before. This is not entirely accurate. On average we haven't had much change in our activity levels since 1980, before the obesity epidemic was here (Westerterp and Speakman, 2008). Of course there are some of us who have less activity, but some of us have more, so this can't be the sole cause of obesity in anyone. As you can see it is real important to watch what goes in much more carefully than what we do to get rid of excess energy. Besides, exercise to burn calories doesn't work right when you do it; instead, exercise should be used to increase your calorie burn even while at rest. Exercise will boost your metabolism. This effectively increases your ability to use that excess body fat for energy even while sitting or sleeping!

Efficient Exercise

The same exercise gives different energy usage for people. Men and women respond differently to exercise. Even the same person may not use the same number of calories doing the same exercise over time. Your body becomes more efficient at doing the same activity with repetition. You waste less motion, breathe slower, or have a lower heart rate during the same exercise. This leads to less energy usage and why it's so hard to exercise off weight. The more you exercise, the better you get at exercising and the less energy you "waste" during exercise. That is why "muscle confusion" or frequently alternating exercises, and high intensity interval training works for many people. Repetitive cardiovascular activities such as jogging, elliptical, and cycling at moderate intensities fail to achieve the body results most people want. There are always exceptions so don't give up if these exercises work for you. Just keep in mind most people don't get results or have very slow results with these aerobic exercises, but some exercise is always better than none.

The most significant results with exercise come from consistency and perseverance. When you incorporate enough activity (walking or climbing stairs) into your daily routine to lose 250 calories per day, you boost your metabolism and can lose as much as twenty-five pounds of fat within the year. Combined with other interventions, the small changes add up over time. Over five years that's 125 pounds of fat loss. By adding adequate water to the exercise, you can boost this to 150 pounds of fat loss over the same five-year period. Meanwhile, you can incorporate other means of shutting off your weight gain triggers to achieve much more.

Building a strong muscular support helps you remain healthy and mobile longer. If you eat well and exercise to build muscle, you will be able to repair your body and resist disease. As you age, you lose muscle mass. Those who maintain their muscle mass will continue to be in good health and live longer, compared to those with lower muscle mass. To fight aging, keep active and eat to maintain your muscle mass.

The places in the world where people live longer are so-called "blue zones," and life expectancy can be fifteen to twenty years more than average. Many attribute it to the diet eaten by the people. Some believe it's a sense of purpose and connection to their community. Others look for magical herbs and foods that alter their health. Research points to the combination of purpose, physical activity, omega-3 rich diet, vegetable intake, and healthy seafood sources of protein as the keys to the longevity seen in Okinawa, Sardinia, and Costa Rica. I believe it's related to overall lifestyle rather than one magic food. Many of us lack the balance these people have in their lives.

When trying to achieve this balance in your body by eliminating fat, you can reduce your calories too much to get weight loss. Starvation doesn't work. Only a consistent healthy lifestyle will decrease your body fat stores over time and give you better health. Obesity is a multifactorial disease. No one thing causes it in everybody. There is a genetic component, nutritional deficiency, lack of activity, and an addiction component. All of these must be addressed to overcome obesity. You have to improve your nutrition and modify your genes with nutrition and exercise. Use the mental success skills to overcome the addiction as seen in my other book, *Fast-Track Your Health*. This becomes easier once you get rid of the physical cravings by improving your nutrition and get the positive reinforcement of endorphin release when you exercise. The biggest benefit of exercise for weight loss isn't the immediate result, it's the boost to your metabolism. That burns more energy between exercise bouts than during the exercise itself.

Activity and Exercise

Automation has created a great discrepancy between the work we used to do every day and what we do now. Difficult tasks that took the manual labor of dozens of people have been reduced to the supervision by a couple of people over heavy equipment or automated production line. You can regain some of the activity lost in the technological winter by getting outside in the spring.

Exercise and reasonable eating has merit for short-term weight loss goals. While we don't know the long-term impact of these interventions, the failure of weight loss for many people suggests that the benefits go away or become less significant when done incorrectly. Be smart about eating and exercising, particularly since they are interlinked. Learn how to make the best use of your nutrition to get the most from exercise and use exercise to silence your fat genes. More important, use this combination to increase your fat-burning gene activity.

Activity level and exercise have an impact on hunger and appetite. While exercise stimulates hunger, it can also help with appetite. One study demonstrated that people who exercise and restrain eating will feel fuller, and there was an increase in the fullness hormone produced in the small intestine (Martins, 2008).

Exercise increases Peptide YY, the major satiety hormone.

Even subtle changes in activity have a profound effect. Standing periodically and walking around for a few minutes will change how your body responds to meals. Most people believe that what you eat determines what happens to your blood sugar levels. This is the basis of glycemic index-based nutrition, where you track what a particular food does to blood glucose levels. You choose lower glycemic foods to curb the insulin spike associated with fat gain. Exercise and activity are just as important. By walking for a few minutes to break up long periods of inactivity, you can reduce the blood sugar levels of a meal and insulin secretion (Dunstan, 2012). An Australian study showed that a two-minute walking episode every twenty minutes is enough for someone who is overweight (Henson et al., 2016).

Two minutes of walking could be done during a workday when you're stuck at your desk, but what about real exercise? Exercise helps you lose excess body fat, increases conditioning and toning of the body, and makes normal daily activities easier to do. I have three young children who are growing very fast. Periodically I carry one of them to bed when they fall asleep. During a recent trip to Disneyland, I had to carry the oldest for nearly an hour, walking a mile after he exhausted himself at the theme park. Carrying him wouldn't have been possible and would have made me extremely sore the next day if not for conditioning and strength training. My life was easier because of exercise, but not every type gives the same benefits.

Some experts advocate aerobic activity for weight loss, others strength training and anaerobic activity. The recommendations have changed over the years, from aerobic exercises to strength training to high intensity interval training to a combination. Planned strength and interval exercise training with fasting and optimized meal strategies make fat loss happen more rapidly. Regardless of the exercise, consistency is the most important factor to make a difference. Even modest amounts of exercise done consistently over time will result in fat loss.

Fat oxidation (fat burning) during exercise varies by exercise type and intensity. During exercise one of the most efficient ways to burn fat is aerobic activity at between fifty-nine percent and sixty-four percent of maximum oxygen consumption in trained individuals and between forty-seven percent and fifty-two percent of maximum oxygen consumption in the average person (Achten and Jeukendrup, 2004). If we go more or less than this, then fat oxidation drops off. There are a couple of problems with this as a means for fat loss. First, this is a very narrow window in most people and we don't all know our oxygen consumption. Second, this fat burning stops as soon as we stop exercising. Finally, this does little to shape our physique, build muscle, and help with boosting our metabolism.

Milo of Croton, a Greek wrestler, grew his physique by carrying a bull on his shoulders daily from the time it was a calf to when it was full grown. While the animal was small at birth, it gained weight over time, but did not change very much on a daily basis. Milo's strength grew as the calf grew. His body was touted as an example of ideal male physique and compared to Hercules.

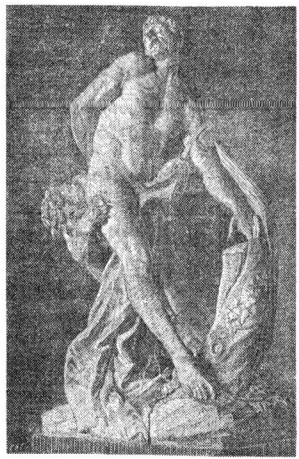

Milo of Croton

You don't have to carry a cow to be in good shape or good health. You only need to get moving and keep moving. A little effort on a regular basis creates a habit that grows over time. When you increase activity, your nutritional demands are increased and you need to eat more. People are often hungrier after working out. This adds up to extra intake. Eat the wrong things and you will be on the road to fat gain even while exercising regularly.

Appetite and Exercise

You can make poor choices if you haven't planned what to eat after exercise, but the bigger problem is when exercise doesn't continue or is sporadic. A UK study showed the increase in appetite and adaptation to increase energy intake continues after you stop exercising (Blundell, 2003). The increased energy intake can be thirty percent of energy expenditure. Even when you burn enough calories through exercise, you will have hunger and eat to gain back the weight. Make good choices about what to eat after exercise and you will come out ahead. When you stop exercising, you stop burning but your appetite doesn't go back to normal for as long as sixteen days.

Assume you normally eat 2600 calories per day. Using an online calorie calculator to figure out how much to reduce your intake to lose a healthy one to two pounds per week, you cut out 400 calories to a daily 2200 calories. Imagine, you exercise vigorously for an hour a day in a spin class and burn 600 calories (based on a 185-pound woman, since people use different energy for the same exercise). Your increased appetite and hunger will cause a thirty percent increase in energy intake, and you eat 780 extra calories above your daily budget of 2200 calories. Soon you are up to 2980 calories per day, or 390 calories more than when you started. At the end of ten days, that 390 extra calories would translate into over a pound of additional fat. Additional weight gain would happen from the stress of daily exercise without appropriate rest and muscle gains. Ten days later, you are actually up three to five pounds from the calories you didn't cut out, the calories you added, and the stress.

This is why weight loss from exercise is hard to maintain. Once you stop, you continue to feel hungry as if you were still exercising regularly. You decrease your energy use for the same exercise by getting more fit and efficient, yet your energy intake remains the same or increases. The problem is your metabolism will slow very quickly once you stop exercising and more if you become deconditioned. Less energy needs and usage at rest is the worst combination. Weight gain can be rapid and why people who were fit soon look fat after stopping exercise.

The choices of what you eat around exercise have a psychological component. Many people think they can control the thirty percent increase in energy uptake, but then the license effect comes into play. When you do something you perceive as healthy, you often give yourself permission, or the license, to do something not so healthy. You can have that burger, candy, or soda because you already worked out. This decision has to be controlled when your exercise does not match the cheat you had. By taking the easy, rewarding choice, you also miss the opportunity to take something better for you.

How Much Exercise?

Not enough exercise is a problem when trying to lose weight. How much you should do is a common question. Some people only want to do as much as necessary to maintain their weight and others want a higher level of fitness. These require different levels of commitment. The threshold for activity to achieve balance is simple to track. The tipping point between inactive and active is 7,116 steps per day (Shook, 2015). This level gives energy balance but won't achieve weight loss. To get weight loss, the threshold is 10,260 steps per day. These are average numbers so you may require an extra two to three thousand steps to get to your personal threshold of balance, fitness, and weight loss. Most fitness trackers, or an inexpensive pedometer, will help you stay on track.

Cardiovascular exercise burns a lot of energy and is great for blood flow and heart conditioning. The problem is this energy is in the form of muscle glycogen and rarely taps into fat stores. Studies show that the energy burning benefits of cardiovascular exercise go away within a couple of hours after stopping, particularly at lower intensities (Bahr, 1991). The more vigorously you exercise the longer the fat-burning benefits you get. What happens when you prolong the exercise, or go long enough to deplete glycogen in muscle and liver? That has to be greater than forty-five minutes to an hour and a half depending on activity level and body mass.

Most people have fat burning machinery that is shut off so you can't easily access your fat stores for energy. This translates to energy deficiency during exercise, which causes muscle breakdown. Access to fat stores is an ability that needs to be developed and supported over time. Your body tries to keep your weight steady. Keeping body conditions steady is called homeostasis. If you have a manic push to exercise and lose fat, you often see it come back on when you can't maintain the same level of commitment. What happens when you push too hard, too fast?

Too much exercise can be stressful and wear you down. It can burn muscle instead of fat and result in slowing your metabolism further. Have you seen people who run on the treadmill, ride their bike, or do spin classes or another form of cardiovascular exercise every day without changing the shape of their bodies significantly? They drag through hours of grueling exercise only to find they get more conditioned but have no external signs it's doing them any good. Or they make significant progress at the beginning to see things stall out months into the process. Excessive exercise leads to muscle burning and fat retention due to stress and lack of coordination with nutrition.

There is nothing more demoralizing than trying to get fit and seeing your body fat stay the same despite your extraordinary effort. This is extremely common. Everyone trying to get fit and lose fat goes through this at some point, but there is a fix on the game. Use the following key concepts that relate to the seasonal character of weight gain and activity to take the next leap forward. Let's start with why the cardiovascular exercise does no good.

Worse than wasting time is the fact that as you increase your aerobic exercise, you have diminishing returns and increased stress on your body. This can lead to adrenal depletion, chronic fatigue, and hormone imbalances (Brooks, 2013). Since a large part of muscular and athletic development relies on your hormonal state, this is disastrous for someone trying to lose weight or be a competitive athlete. Prolonged daily workouts along with chronic stress, perfectionism, poor eating, shiftwork, or any of those in combination and other stressors can lead to chronic fatigue from adrenal insufficiency. More isn't always better.

While bone density in limbs may increase with running, lumbar spine bone density is lower due to high mileage and overtraining

(MacKelvie, 2000). Lumbar spine stress contributes to low back pain. Does aerobic exercise, endurance training, or running sound appealing right now?

Muscle Mass

Strength training works by a much different process. By building muscle mass, you increase your ongoing energy demands and use up sugars regularly. You also call for fat conversion to sugar by gluconeogenesis in the liver.

Exercise stimulates gluconeogenesis within the liver to make more sugar fuel for muscles by breaking down fat.

Strength training burns energy in the short-term but at slightly slower rates than cardiovascular exercise. The difference is muscle-building activity results in high-energy use for two to three days after the exercise stops. This makes your overall energy usage for strength exercise greater than cardiovascular exercise. Some people refute this and any other benefit of certain exercise types because no populations or methods for calculating benefit are the same. The length of time, population, body type, nutrition, season, temperature, and many other factors play a role in how energy is used during exercise. These are general principles for most people trying to gain muscle and lose fat.

One method is to exercise like a child. When a child runs a race, they bolt and hold nothing back. They go until they can't go any more and then stop, rest, and go again with bursts of energy. Most people try to save energy for later. You have experienced being tired—you dread it and try to conserve energy by sitting, walking, and slowing down overall. Give every moment the attention it deserves and the energy it takes to perform at your peak. Saving nothing for later is how children operate. Animals never think about saving energy. They do what is necessary for the activity at hand. This is just like high intensity interval training (HIIT). Chasing food, climbing a tree, or escaping predators require energy usage and it doesn't make sense to save energy for later. As humans, we rarely worry about survival any more. Those who have to survive their environment generally thin down. They eat and stay active just to survive.

Many exercise experts, health coaches, and dietary experts suggest eating and exercising like an animal. While this seems unusual, this is more in tune with your natural instincts and similar to the creatures in the wild that are never overweight. Like seasonal changes in diet, animals have a lot to teach us. The stress that comes with life being out of your control contributes more to your weight gain and poor health than the lack of healthy nutrition and exercise. Regain some control through understanding of how nature intended you to eat and exercise.

High Intensity Interval Training

Not all stored calories in your body are easy to access. First goes the glycogen in your muscles, followed by the glycogen in your liver. Finally, you access fat. Most people can do almost two hours of exercise before running out of glycogen. This is the "wall" you hit when running long distances. But do you have two hours to spend getting to fat burning, and exercising beyond that to burn the fat? Three hours of exercise is too much and you're likely busy enough in your life, not to mention the risk of over exercising.

The scientific literature shows the tricks for getting over this biological hurdle and activating the genes that engage your fat burning machinery. Are you ready for a lot of free time? Write a schedule for the goals you want to achieve and chores around the house because the time you save with the advice I share should be put to good use or you might spend it on weight-gaining activities.

High intensity interval training (HIIT) is how to go. Unless you are devoting your life to exercise or becoming a professional level athlete, hours of training are not what you need to get the most out of exercise. Many competitive athletes use some of these same techniques to get a scientific advantage in their gains. You will get fit faster but there are no short cuts to making your body look like a movie star. Nutrition and other factors are eighty to eighty-five percent of weight loss and exercise only accounts for fifteen to twenty percent of improvement. So, get the most out of it. Scientific studies show you can compress exercise into shorter bouts of high intensity activity and make gains greater than moderate intensity activity. Not only is aerobic capacity improved by thirteen percent, but anaerobic capacity increased by twenty-eight percent in a six-week study period (Tabata, 1996). You can gain a thirteen percent improvement in your ability to carry out aerobic activity such as running, biking, or swimming, and the equivalent of twenty-eight percent more power and strength in activities like weight lifting.

What does this mean for you? Suppose you jog for thirty minutes as your daily exercise—how can you make this more effective? Shorten it to eight minutes and you gain twenty-two minutes to prepare a healthy meal with a good balance of carbohydrates, protein, and healthy fats. Here's how to spend the eight minutes exercising: for the first minute, sprint as fast as you can. Pretend a large dog, lion, or bear is chasing you—whatever motivates you to move like the wind. Only do this for a minute. Rest for the next minute, sprint for a minute, rest for a minute, and so forth until your eight minutes are up. The time you run seems like an eternity and the rest breaks are too short. You might start with fewer sets early on. It really is challenging.

Make it better by going in one direction for slightly more than half the time and return to your starting point in the remaining time—this forces yourself to go faster. The same principle can be used in walking, swimming, and bicycling. Pick the exercise compatible with your level of fitness and which you enjoy. For bicycling, do twenty-second sprints with a twenty-second recovery, the same with swimming. You want to be exhausted by these sprints. The HIIT literature suggests seven to eight sets, but you can start at fewer and work up higher as your abilities improve (Tabata et al., 1996). Once you get to ten sets, reduce the recovery to half. For example, run one minute, rest thirty seconds, bike twenty seconds, and rest ten seconds. Continue until you reach a four to one ratio of exercise to rest. By then, you will be doing well at maximizing your results. Start with a one to four exercise to rest ratio if you are out of shape and work to gradually flip those numbers. I'm not suggesting a specific exercise or sport, just giving you the tools to unlock your potential.

Aerobic activity isn't always the most efficient way to gain muscle and lose fat. With the same HIIT principle for muscle building, I use kettlebell exercises with a skilled instructor. This gives the combination of dynamic movements, explosive strength, endurance, and flexibility. My workouts last twenty minutes. I trimmed the last couple of fat inches off my waist with this method and built enough strength to improve my running times and endurance without the endless pounding of the pavement. You can use different exercise methods to get to the same results.

Take a short cut to activating your fat burning signals and get the benefits of a shorter work out by using the techniques above. You can also exercise at the time of day for the most good. The best time is after a prolonged fast, namely when you wake up in the morning and haven't eaten since dinner. At that time, your glycogen stores are naturally depleted (Van Proeyen, 2011). This can provide immediate access to fat stores and boost fat oxidation. Surprisingly, blood sugar levels don't drop during exercise, as you might worry about. Unless you have low blood sugar issues, blood sugar should be steady.

Exercise in the morning is said to provide three hundred percent more fat burning. The real number is approximately twenty-one percent fat burned with fasting compared to six percent with carbohydrates. Three hundred percent comes from comparing the twenty-one percent to the six percent. The numbers are more realistic when you understand what they really are. How does this work? Fasted exercise works by activating a gene that increases mitochondrial energy metabolism. Mitochondria are your power-houses, where you make the energy for your cells to survive.

The gene is called PGC-1a. There is greater than an eight-fold increase in this gene with fasted exercise compared to 2.5 times increase with exercise at normal glycogen levels (after eating).

This useful tool is not the only answer. Fasting is a period without eating and has nothing to do with how much nutrition or calories you take in when you do eat. You still get your caloric and nutritional requirements during the time you are eating. This is unlike the drastic dieting where overall calories and nutrition decrease for a prolonged time. In that situation the body is stripped of nutrition and increases the activation of fat storing genes.

Get Active and Stay Active

Every day you experience positive and negative situations. Sometimes it's easy to fall into constant thought about an unpleasant experience and this sticks with you for a while. Fear extinction means a particular fear is gone. You've gotten over it. Many people think of fear as phobias, but you have fear all the time, like confronting people at work, dealing with your teenage children, or doing work that makes you uncomfortable. Each of these trigger fear to an extent. When you are constantly eating and then go hungry, this prevents fear extinction from happening. In contrast, when you fast during a period where you experience a fear-inducing event, the fear disappears quickly (Verma, 2016). You can use your hunger genes not only to lose fat, but also to get rid of fear and anxiety. When you put hunger together with exercise, you gain physical benefits and your fear of exercise quickly dissipates as well.

Exercise signals your muscle cells' DNA to produce key substances that help with weight loss. These include testosterone, growth hormone, and several others. Each improves fat loss and muscle gain, and together they are an unstoppable force for improving your health (Miller, 2012; Wideman, 2002). Some of these substances are a solution to fat loss, muscle building, and anti-aging. Your body's ability to boost them comes without the risks or complications when taking a drug or synthetic form.

Good nutrition and activity provides the right nutrients and the right stimulus so you can harness the power of these amazing hormones for fat burning and muscle building DNA. Fat genes are inactivated by methylation, and the opposite happens to your muscle building genes after exercise (Barrès, 2012). They are demethylated, or activated. Exercise changes which genes are turned on. The more intense the exercise, the higher substances like growth hormone get in your body regardless of age. You can build muscle, burn fat, and feel fit at any age.

Getting active and restoring these substances in your body while activating fat burning happens one step at a time. Keeping track of your food intake makes sure you get all of your nutrients on a regular basis, and tracking your exercise ensures you stick to it. Maintaining consistency ensures your progress doesn't stagnate or put you at risk for injury or fatigue. Enjoy the activity and include others with you. Turn it into game play. You will get fit, feel better, and have fun as you take control of your health.

Here is a list of activities that turn on your fat burning genes:

1. Start with regular daily small amounts of exercise
2. High intensity interval training (HIIT) activates muscle building and fat burning faster
3. Nutrition to support muscle building, including adequate protein several hours before exercise and shortly after exercise
4. Healthy fats to support muscle building and recovery
5. Fasted exercise to maximize fat burning
6. Graduated increases in exercise intensity to prevent injury and continue gains
7. Exercise in the morning before breakfast

Just as important as exercise is making sure you recognize the stress it causes to your body. Make sure you eat and supplement appropriately to recover. Don't overdo it. Remember, there is a point of diminishing returns in exercise. More isn't always better for the regular person or an athlete. There is a risk of strain, injury, and worsening performance from stress. Consider stress and fatigue when you decide on how much exercise to do and how long it takes to recover.

❄ 12

Catching Cold, Catching Fat

The common cold has been associated with weight gain in animals (Voss, 2015), and cold virus exposure can increase the risk of obesity in people as well. Since no experiment has proven anything more than an association, there is little proof that the common cold makes you fat. Infecting a bunch of people with the virus to see if they get fatter is ethically wrong, but animal studies and the association show this is true. As the human population rises and more time is spent indoors, the risk for catching infections from each other increases.

Adenovirus 36 is the specific cold virus shown, among others, to contribute to weight gain over time.

The need for more sources of food has grown along with the population. Increased meat production and larger congregations of pigs and fowl are the perfect breeding grounds for new viral infections that drive weight gain, appetite, and food demand. Viruses that cause us to gain weight are a clever evolutionary survival mechanism. Just like other signals from the environment that tell us a hardship is coming, such as the temperature or the nutrients in food, your body is programmed to defend against viruses.

All of the contacts and interactions make transmitting those awful little germs difficult to avoid. The greater number of people, the more likely you are to be infected, and the number of exposures to different viruses increases. What else happens when many animals are stuck in a small area? They compete for food. Your body has the ability to store fat when the competition for food gets too intense.

It detects this through the outside signals of infections as well as the quality and quantity of nutrition you take in. Exposing your body to more infections increases the signaling. Decrease the food intake or quality and your body responds. We can't abandon society and run into the mountains to escape virus-induced weight gain but we can help this problem. Here are a few simple things that can reverse the signaling of competition:

1. Avoid crowded indoor areas during the cold and flu season
2. Wash your hands before eating or touching your eyes, nose, or mouth
3. Maintain good nutrition, and take plenty of vitamins (antioxidant source) and minerals that allow your body to detect good nutrition and defend against infection
4. Avoid processed food with lots of processed fats that interfere with immunity
5. No matter what you think or have heard, get immunized

Other Causes for Weight Gain

Certain bacteria, viruses, and even yeast are linked to obesity or been causative factors. Surprisingly, the same foods that drive weight-gain can provide nutrition for viruses and keep them growing. This puts you at higher risk for weight gain, inflammation, and other problems. Over one hundred trillion bacteria are in the human body, and the number of human cells is between ten and thirty trillion. Bacteria outnumber your human cells by ten to one. This doesn't include viral counts or yeast. If many of the bacteria are bad, you can end up being hijacked into bad health.

Ninety-nine percent of the DNA or genes in your body belongs to the bacteria. With the knowledge about gene modification by exposure, you should be able to control which bacteria you have in your gut, train that bacteria to turn on the genes you want, while shutting down their ability to make you fat. Many of the solutions to turning off your fat genes work the same way on bacteria.

There is a lot of hidden information about how your body deals with stress and danger and how you use energy at those times and after in anticipation of new dangers. Does your body's bacterial environment have an impact on health and weight? Is this microbiome (the bacteria on and in your body) affected by what you eat or not spending time in the sun? Does what you eat have an impact on your ability to resist infections? It's important to know the answers to the many questions on this subject. They hold natural secrets to why people gain weight.

Your Weight and the Microbiome

The microbiome is a unique combination for every human being, like your fingerprint. Families in the same household and eating the same foods have similar microbiomes. Let's take a look at the impact this has on your weight.

An interesting study highlighted the question of what role do bacteria in our gut play in weight gain (Liou, 2013). Scientists experimented on obese animals and performed weight loss surgery to achieve a healthy weight. Along with the weight loss, the bacteria in the animal's stools changed significantly. It might seem obvious that when you change your food intake it changes the bacteria, but the scientists delved into what was behind the change and what significance it might have. The new bacteria from the animals with surgery were transplanted to obese animals without surgery, and they lost weight too. While the bacteria were thought to be a side effect of the surgery, perhaps the effect of the surgery was due to the change in the bacteria. This might be caused by the surgery itself or the change in eating habits of those who had weight loss surgery. With increased healthy foods and decreased intake of refined foods (starches and sugars), there was less for the bad bacteria to consume.

In people, this change happens in the microbiome with fat gain (Quigley, 2013) and again after weight loss surgery (Kong, 2013).

The bacteria between people who are overweight and those of normal weight are very different. Bacteria play a huge role in our health and the development of obesity, type 2 diabetes, and insulin resistance (Molinaro, 2012). The changes don't just happen in animals, but in you. The type of bacteria you ingest (probiotics) has a significant impact on weight loss (Bjerg, 2014; Sanchez, 2014). The wrong bacteria in your gut and antibiotics that kill the good bacteria will increase the rate of weight gain. This happens by signals from the bacteria to increase fat storage. The type of bacteria makes you more efficient at extracting energy from food (Aguirre, 2014). It also makes sense that other types of bacteria can activate your DNA to slow down energy absorption or return it to normal.

The problem is that the bacteria don't change by themselves. Reliance on antibiotics and treatments that eradicate bacteria are partially to blame. For example, *H. pylori* (*Helicobacter pylori*) is a bacteria found in the stomach, which has been associated with ulcer disease. Its treatment became the recommended standard of care in the 1990s for people suffering from ulcers—and this expanded to anyone with unexplained upper abdominal pain. Treating bad bacteria that cause ulcers makes sense, but was the overgrowth of *H. pylori* and the ulcer disease cause and effect or just an association? That question is still being answered and the negative result is that people who have been treated for *H. pylori* also gained weight (Dhurandhar, 2015). Fantastic choice: either you get ulcer disease or you get fat. Let me suggest a better alternative.

The types of foods you eat have an impact on the type of bacteria as well. Some foods cause microorganisms like bad bacteria and yeast to grow, while others promote different healthier varieties. Reversing the process of bacteria-induced weight gain involves getting the right types of bacteria in place through changes in diet, dynamic changes in the gut environment through weight loss surgery, and addition of probiotics. This field is still in development, as proven by the large numbers of patients that choose deforming intestinal surgeries as the solution. Most of them, including their doctors, don't know that part of what they are doing is affecting the microbiome. If they did, alternative treatments would be added to increase weight loss before resorting to surgery or improve outcomes after surgery.

Using the same ulcer example, you can manipulate the nutrients and bacteria you get to reverse the damage done by the overgrowth of *H. pylori* or the results of treatment. Recent studies are looking into doing this with combinations of probiotics, omega-3 fats, and plant-based treatments (Homan, 2015; Han, 2015). Taking a harmless *Lactobacillus* probiotic may eliminate the need for the inconvenient and expensive antibiotics and antacids used for years. *Lactobacillus* is cheaper, potentially more effective, and has the added benefit of weight loss instead of weight gain.

Unfortunately, obesity disease still carries a stigma, inferring that its cause is laziness or lack of self-control. As you see, many factors contribute to weight gain. This does not absolve you from the responsibility of making good choices, improving your health, and avoiding as many weight-gain triggers as possible. A balance must be struck between identifying the biological processes of weight gain and ensuring habitual issues are addressed. This is like addiction medicine because of the diet-induced rewards for poor choices. These can be overcome, especially if you set the stage with good nutrition, proper information, appropriate medical advice, and planned interventions.

In the future, the type of gut flora will determine who gets what kind of treatment for obesity since the flora has been linked to successful response in dietary intervention (Korpela, 2014). Changing to normal flora will help return you to normal weight. More treatments will be geared toward changing the bacteria in your gut to those that encourage health and leaner body types. We have seen an explosion in probiotics containing active bacterial species as a supplement or in yogurt. Other sources of useful bacteria are around the corner.

There're specific bacteria already studied that have a potential for increasing fat loss. For instance, one study monitored the use of a certain probiotic in women trying to lose weight. The results were astonishing. Women taking the bacterium as a probiotic along with a healthy diet had 120 percent greater fat loss over a six-month period than those only eating healthy (Sanchez, 2014), creating a more than ten-pound difference. Another probiotic was found to suppress appetite without affecting insulin or glucose (Bjerg, 2014). This suggests that these passengers in your body have a huge impact on what happens in your belly and brain. These angels on the head of the pin can either lead you toward health or be the devils that lead you to weight gain and illness.

Other bacteria have shown similar results for weight loss (Kadooka, 2010). Some bacteria do the opposite. You don't want to get the wrong probiotics on board. A common species of bacteria found in many yogurt probiotics has been found to actually cause weight gain (Million, 2012). It's not about gulping down any probiotics. You have to use the right ones.

Probiotics that help weight loss include: Lactobacillus rhamnosus, Lactobacillus paracasei, and Lactobacillus gasseri. The common Lactobacillus acidophilus (or just acidophilus) is a weight gain probiotic.

Healthy bacteria can reduce obesity and reverse the dietary toxins that cause obesity. Studies of MSG-induced obesity show a reversal by adding a probiotic (Savcheniuk, 2014). It's not just about losing weight. The same study demonstrated decreased triglycerides and bad cholesterol (LDL), with an increase in good cholesterol (HDL). Along with these improvements is also the loss of visceral fat, the internal fat around your organs that increases your risk for disease.

More recently, prebiotics have become popular. Not only do we want healthy bacteria but we also want the right types of foods to support that good bacteria's growth. Prebiotics are foods that support healthy bacterial flora in your gut. These foods provide food for the bacteria. If you starve your bacteria, you will be right back where you started. Healthy bacteria plus healthy food equals a healthy gut, digestion, and body.

Recently research has shown that viruses actually are more numerous in our bodies and gut than bacteria. The gut bacteria may be a way that we keep these in check. Just imagine we have ten times the number of bacterial cells as our own cells and maybe as much as hundred times that in viruses! A balance in these, having the right ones and eliminating the bad becomes even more important as we learn more about their relationship to our health and weight.

For years the focus has been on just eliminating bacteria and germs, yet now we know they are necessary and may be the key to the good health you are looking for. Rather than avoiding or treating a disease, look for what you can do to promote health. Taking probiotics with healthy bacteria is one, eating natural foods is another, making sure you get enough fiber to support a healthy colon where most of our bacteria lives is yet another; and finally making sure you avoid, prevent, and recover well from viral infections is just as important.

Toxins in Your Environment

Chemicals affect your health, brain, body, and behavior. Not only do they determine how you feel but also how you act. How does this happen? Chemical additives to food, pesticides, plastics, and other substances in your daily life have an impact on how your body works. They can turn on or turn off certain genes and cell functions. Some of these have been implicated in weight gain and other diseases. Just like sugar acts like a neurotoxin, other environmental substances can act as toxins and have impact on your health. Toxins must either be eliminated or reduced.

Certain dietary components act as neurotoxins causing brain dysfunction that can be measured cognitively. The problem is not just that your brain doesn't work as well but you end up making poor choices. This leads to poor food choices and taking in more of the same toxin—another vicious cycle that contributes to weight gain. Other foods protect the brain and block the effects of these toxins. Other than plain white sugar, the major implicated toxin to the brain is fructose, as in high fructose corn syrup (HFCS). This is in everything and manufacturers have now started removing HFCS because of public backlash. In experiments, fructose causes reduction in mental capabilities (Agrawal, 2012). Animals exposed to HFCS can't complete tasks they had learned before. Teachers have experienced this with their students requiring more effort to learn or having less retention than in the past. It is no wonder since most of our so-called breakfast foods contain either sugar or HFCS.

It's naive to believe the effect of HFCS is localized to only one type of neuron in the brain. HFCS affects neurons throughout the brain including the hypothalamus. The hypothalamus is the central control area of the brain. This helps explain why some people who continue to gain weight have difficulty regulating their body temperature and why some people feel hotter than before they gained weight.

It's not just HFCS, but all refined sugar does this. If we compare sugar as a snack to, say, protein or lecithin (a fatty substance containing choline derived from egg yolks and other foods) we find that brain function declines with the sugar and improves with the other nutrients. When the sugar is taken away the brain returns to normal. The lecithin and protein give the opposite effect (Meck and Church, 1987). Unfortunately, when we are tired or want to focus what do we reach for? I bet you have reached for a sugary beverage with caffeine. If you've been watching commercials, maybe you reach for a candy bar? Perhaps an egg, some nuts, or a cup of milk might have been better?

Protein and fat seem to have improved brain function when taken and one type of fat in particular seems to top them all. Omega-3 fatty acids completely reverse the brain dysfunction that results from HFCS. These have become a popular supplement for weight loss because they counteract the negative effects of HFCS and have other benefits for health and weight loss. Omega-3 deficiency causes the disruption of cell membrane homeostasis, or the ability to regulate cell function, detection of environmental stimulus by cells, and regulation of movement of materials across the membrane. This is extremely dangerous, considering that the membrane is the means of communication between one cell and the next, and how the cell detects and defends against toxins. The membrane can detect environmental substances that stimulate weight gain called "obesogens."

Weight Gain by Obesogens

Many substances contribute to obesity, some by altering how fat is burned while others stimulate you to eat more. Still others mimic sex hormones. All these substances change how your genes are expressed or activated. Some of them are well known and easily avoidable while others require more thought and planning to eliminate. There are over twenty known obesogens and more uncovered daily. Additives in food, including soy and monosodium glutamate, have also been linked to weight gain.

Bisphenol A (BPA) is derived from plastics and epoxy and shows up in many places you wouldn't expect. For instance, aluminum soda cans are lined with plastic or epoxy to keep the acid in the soda from reacting with the metal. Just sitting there, some of the materials from the epoxy will end up in the liquid. When that soda can heats in the sun, BPA leaches out of the epoxy faster. Plastic water bottles are one of the most common sources of this obesity-causing substance. Whenever plastic is exposed to high heat such as in the sun, low temperatures such as in the refrigerator or freezer, or detergents such as in the dishwasher, BPA is released. Animal studies with BPA show that it disrupts genomic imprinting—which is how your genetic code chooses between dad's or mom's genes.

BPA, atrazine and DDE (dichlorodiphenyldichloroethylene—a DDT breakdown product), and even certain medications have been linked to increased BMI. Medications, like the diabetes drug Avandia® (rosiglitazone), have been linked to weight.

The component of soy that mostly contributes to weight gain is the soy phytoestrogen genistein.

BPA is a synthetic estrogen analogue that mimicks the hormone estrogen and can cause increase weight gain and increased risk for breast cancer.

Genomic imprinting is definitely a term that requires a definition. You get two copies of each of your genes from your parents. Genomic imprinting is how the body decides to turn on one versus the other of the genes. Certain environmental factors affect genes from mother or father differently and turn on one or the other set. If your mother's genes contribute more to your weight and are turned on, your risk of obesity will be higher. If your father has high blood pressure and you turn on the genes from him, your risk of high blood pressure will go up.

BPA has been shown to disrupt genomic imprinting in mice and cause problems with placental development and early fetal development. The placenta is how the baby connects to its mother through the umbilical cord. Obviously, you get higher risk for an abnormal baby if the placenta doesn't develop normally to support the developing fetus. BPA activates one of the obesity genes (Susiarjo, 2013). Female mice given BPA during pregnancy gave birth to litters of blond mice who went on to develop obesity, diabetes, heart disease, and cancers and died an early death. Sound familiar?

We have an epidemic growing out of control. How bad is BPA for people? Girls with elevated BPA levels are twice as likely to be obese then those with low BPA levels (Li, 2013).

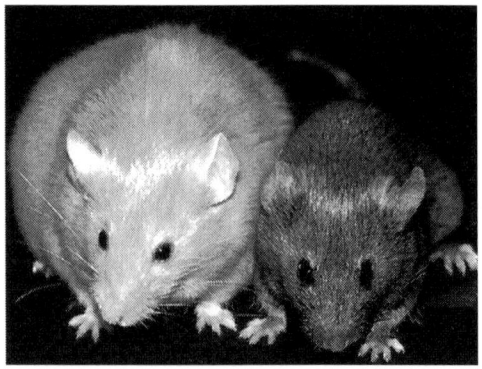

Just like the bad genes can be turned on, they can be turned off again too. Your fate is not set in stone. The scientists that observed the changes in mice with BPA theorized that by giving the mothers methyl donors (foods that contribute methyl groups that can be attached to their DNA such as garlic and onions) they could deactivate the bad gene (Dolinoy, 2007). Methylation, the addition of methyl groups to DNA, turns off those genes. When the same mouse mother that was fed BPA during pregnancy was also fed methyl donors during her pregnancy, her offspring came out normal in size and color. The difference between the fat, blond, unhealthy mouse and the skinny, healthy brown mouse show how changing the mother's diet can make a difference and lead to healthier mice. The skinny mouse had none of the risks for diabetes, heart disease, or cancers and lived a full, healthy life. That's a huge difference in appearance and in health in genetically identical mice just based on mom's exposures during pregnancy.

The increasing frequency of medical conditions seen in people across the U.S. and around the world is mimicked in this experiment. Just like the mice, human mothers can affect their unborn children's risk of these conditions and so can the father. Just as important we can use these same methods to modify the risk from toxins we are exposed to and shut off the unhealthy genes.

Plastics Contribute to Obesity

You just heard about one substance from plastics, BPA, that contributes to obesity but that's just the tip of the iceberg. Dioxin exposure from plastics has received much press as a possible cause of cancer and a potential contributor to obesity (Kim, 2012; Arsenescu, 2008). Dioxin comes from plastic but also from natural sources such as certain foods and flavorings. Studies have found that allowing food to burn or cooking with certain foods causes dioxin production. Foods that contain high amounts of organic chlorine produce dioxins when cooked. This can occur naturally or from environmental contamination. Cattle, chicken, and seafood concentrate environmental pollutants from the food they eat. The contamination is usually in the fat. Organically raised meats are better because they are less likely to be exposed to these contaminants. Marinating meats with onion, garlic, and other spices will reduce the production of dioxin during the cooking process. Marinating isn't just about tenderizing meat or adding flavor, it is also about reducing the damage the food will do when you eat it. However, it's not only the food we have to be careful of. The smoke or vapors from cooking also carry dioxin (Wu, 2011). Having good ventilation during cooking is important for preventing inhalation of this material.

So far, we have looked at two toxins that come from plastics. The question I always get next is, "What if I use BPA-free items?" Many other chemical pollutants come from plastics, even BPA-free plastics. The irony is some of the BPA-free plastics release even more toxic substances. How many toxins are we exposed to? Hundreds, and possibly thousands, of toxins leach out of plastics including the ones already mentioned. Many of these are known to have harmful hormone-mimicking effects that lead to obesity. The problem with testing the effects of these substances on people is that they are reported to be present in amounts smaller than a "toxic" dose as defined by the government. Besides, it would be unethical to do an experiment where you're giving a toxin to people to see the result. The aforementioned population studies have shown the effects of toxins on obesity and other health problems; we just need to repeat them for these other substances.

Despite the evidence, the Food and Drug Administration (FDA) amazingly has come out saying that BPA is not dangerous. The studies have also shown that combinations of toxins cause more harm than any individual toxin. It is not unusual to see contradictory information about specific, individual toxins. When the FDA looks at a study of only one toxin, it is difficult for them to come to a conclusion about the toxicity of that substance since the levels of most normal exposures are low.

Repeated exposure to poor diet, exercise, heat, and toxins can have an impact greater than just a single exposure but what happens when you have exposure to multiple toxins at the same time repeatedly? Do they cause more harm? Is their effect additive? The great dilemma is how to evaluate this and what to do with plastics that have become ubiquitous in our society. Even canned goods have plastic toxins in them. Metal cans are lined with thin layers of plastic or epoxy to make them last longer. Before this change in manufacturing, canned goods were usually packaged in steel cans so the worst that would happen was more iron in your diet, providing that the steel manufacturing process didn't contain contaminant heavy metals. Now you get neither the potential benefit of steel cans nor are you protected from the harm of plastics. Worse, we have been exposed to full plastic and aluminum containers as alternatives to steel and glass containers driven by cheaper manufacturing costs and decreased shipping costs of container materials.

MSG and Other Dangers

Monosodium glutamate (MSG) is sometimes referred to as yeast extract, hydrolyzed vegetable protein, or textured vegetable protein. It is usually used as a flavoring for foods. If you have ever eaten food high in MSG you might notice feeling very thirsty, having your hands or feet swell, or eating more than you normally would. But what else is going on? The same MSG used to flavor your food creates obesity in rats. Since we don't eat the same diet or have the same lifestyle it's hard to show how this happens in people. In rats, their handlers control feedings, making it very easy to prove. The MSG affects the hunger center of the brain and sets off a hunger response. It makes you eat more, and that's why it's put in food in the first place.

The hunger center affected by MSG is in the arcuate nucleus of the brain.

Medications can also contribute to significant weight gain. People with unhealthy lifestyle or a family history of elevated cholesterol may be put on statin medications to help lower cholesterol and presumably the risk of stroke and heart disease. These medications have the unfortunate side effect of causing increased weight gain. This creates another vicious circle of worsening health and more medications that add to the weight gain. In fact, the same studies that demonstrated improved cardiac risk with statins also showed those using these medications are twenty-seven percent more likely to develop diabetes than those not using them (Shah, 2012). Diabetes is usually treated with insulin or medications—both of which cause more weight gain. Can you see how frustrating this process becomes?

Pesticides are another group of pollutants that have an impact on health. These often mimic hormones in their structure or function. They interfere with an insect's metabolism, effectively killing them. Unfortunately, they affect us too. According to food producers, nutrient content between organically grown and foods grown using pesticides is identical. Any difference should be attributable to the pesticide residues on them. Let's assume for a moment the food producers are right and the only difference is the residues. How dangerous can these be? It's only a little bit. We wash our fruits and vegetables, and that's enough, isn't it? Apparently not.

A study from Norway looked at the eating habits of over 28,000 pregnant women, comparing the incidence of preeclampsia among those who ate organic produce most of the time versus those who didn't (Torjusen, 2014). Preeclampsia is a serious complication of pregnancy where the mother's blood pressure is high and she gets kidney dysfunction, liver dysfunction, and low platelet counts, and much more. The baby is at the risk of being born prematurely and has a higher risk of death. The mothers eating organic food most of the time had an almost forty percent less risk of developing preeclampsia. Imagine knowing that eating a certain way can reduce the risk of a disease by 40%! Pesticide residues are so toxic that they result in at least forty percent more pregnancy complications. Right from the start, we are put at risk from the food our mother eats.

How do pesticide residues affect obesity? A study was done looking at polychlorinated biphenyls (PCB), a pesticide residue, in over 12,000 people. Those with higher exposures to pesticides were almost sixty percent more likely to become obese over the eight-year period (Donat-Vargas, 2014). This was after controlling for differences in energy intake. You must be wondering why I didn't put that in all caps, italic, bold, and with exclamation points. The only reason I didn't was because I was too stunned when I read the article to punctuate properly.

The question has changed from "Do these substances have an impact on our weight?" to "How can we continue to allow them?" If you have struggled with weight or have weight issues in your family, shouldn't you be taking action to reduce your risk? By eliminating these substances from your individual food supply, you drive demand for cleaner, less contaminated food. This in turn will bring down costs as more farmers produce untainted food. Right now organic produce is at a premium. This is driven by lower supply. When you think about it, the labor for spraying, and the use of synthetic fertilizers and pesticides are a large portion of production costs, but there are extra labor and costs associated with organic farming. Organic foods are subject to spoiling faster because they have achieved their ripeness and maturity naturally. These foods have to be distributed and eaten quickly. This means we need faster distribution or local production. This again can reduce costs and make the process not only more efficient, but also more affordable.

Careful washing of fruits and vegetables will remove some of the surface residues, and combination of vinegar and lemon juice removes even more. Unfortunately, absorbed toxins within the fruits and vegetables can't be eliminated with washing since they are inside. Cleaning can be inconvenient and difficult to do on the run. Eating organic fruits and vegetables is safer for this reason. Regular produce is cheaper, because it is harder to clean and carries a higher risk to the consumer.

Air pollution is an increasing risk. We think it has no impact on our health other than maybe adding to respiratory symptoms. Evidence to the contrary has started to appear, with studies showing the impact on blood glucose levels (Sade, 2015). The risk is even greater for diabetics. As if there wasn't enough affecting your blood sugar, here is another. The same substances causing acid rain and global warming increase your chances of diabetes.

Emulsifiers are added to foods to give them an even texture throughout. These substances act like detergents and can irritate the intestine, cause digestive problems and inflammation, and set off weight gain (Cani, 2015).

Milk was already mentioned as a potential contributor for weight gain if taken in excess but let's look at some interesting facts about why. First, it is a high-fat, high-protein, sugary fluid designed to give baby cows enough energy and materials to live and grow. When taken in moderation it can help human children do the same. It provides a source of whey protein, which has been found to help maintain muscle mass, as well as being a source of vitamin D and calcium. Even without added hormones, milk may contain microRNAs (mRNAs) that boost expression of one of the fat genes (Melnik, 2015). Use organic milk in moderation to reduce contamination and reduce the risk of excessive mRNAs.

Damaging Processes and Detoxification

Three chemical processes damage your body from normal things you eat and exposures from the environment. These include glycation, oxidation, and inflammation. Most people are familiar with inflammation and oxidation and while these contribute to obesity, I want to touch on the third process, glycation.

Glycation happens when there is production of substances called advance glycation end-products (AGEs). These form when sugars bind to the amino acids in proteins and damage them. This is the conclusion of a multi-stage process that can be reversed. The glycation process happens inside the body or during food preparation. The problem with AGEs is that they can bind to the surface of cells, resulting in damage like premature aging of the skin, atherosclerosis, kidney disease, and diabetes. High sugar content in meals can result in glycation in the body. The damage to cell surfaces and the ability of these AGEs to bind to low-density lipoprotein (LDL) cholesterol, the bad cholesterol, means the surface of cells in blood vessels and the cholesterol become stickier. They bind to each other and result in plaque formation in the vessels. The damage to the muscle proteins means loss of muscle, or, in the case of blood vessels, stiffening of the arterial walls.

Glycation also happens when you process food with cooking. Types of food and method of preparation can lead to increase in AGEs. The browning from fried or baked foods is the production of some AGEs. Dry heat in cooking can result in ten to one hundred times the AGEs as cooking with moist heat. Animal foods high in fat and protein are AGEs rich. Vegetables, fruits, and grains as well as milk have fewer AGEs. You can reduce these AGEs with shorter cooking time, moist heat, decreased temperature, and adding acidic ingredients (Uribarri, 2010). There are increased markers of oxidative stress when you increase exposure to AGEs, and cause **oxidation** and **inflammation.**

How do you detoxify from these pollutants? The liver plays a large role in eliminating toxins from the body. The problem is that the liver is important for weight loss as well. If the liver is overwhelmed with toxins, this can interfere with fat metabolism. This has been known for more than thirty-five years. Alcohol is one toxin that interferes with fat metabolism and causes additional storage of fat in the liver (Baraona, 1979). When the liver stores fat and you have a poor diet, you are more likely to store additional fat because the liver can't handle the excess energy intake.

Conversely, if you overwhelm the liver with fat storage and don't have the proper nutrition for liver health, you can interfere with detoxification of toxins you are exposed to. The liver detoxifies the food you eat and the substances you are exposed to in two phases. The first phase turns toxic substances into less toxic substances.

The first phase involves the P450 system of enzymes to detoxify toxins in the body. This also works on some medications.

Phase two is where toxic substances are bound to a vehicle to make them easy to eliminate from the body by making them water-soluble. This is through urine, sweat, or stool. Ironically, the same substances and toxins that the liver helps detoxify can overwhelm the liver and cause excess fat storage that stores more of the toxins and interferes with the detoxification. Many fat-storing contaminants are things we are commonly exposed to in developed and developing countries. In North America, these substances not only have effects on storing fat in the liver but also in changing how cholesterol moves in the body (Mailloux, 2014).

Generally, the liver is the first place you gain or lose fat. Excess fat in the liver can cause inflammation, lead to fatty liver disease or steatohepatitis, cirrhosis of the liver, and ultimately liver failure. Fat storage in the liver also leads to diabetes. It takes time to lose the excess fat from the liver, almost a month or more depending on the severity of the fat storage, diet, and activity levels. Most of the damage to the liver is reversible. You usually don't see outward signs of weight loss early on because the liver is in the abdomen and hides behind the rib cage on the right. After losing a few pounds in a month, there are no noticeable outward changes. The frustration causes many people to slide back to old habits and overeat to comfort themselves because they feel their efforts have been in vain.

You are about to start making an impact on your health at this point. It's like digging for gold and stopping a foot from the mother lode. Don't do it. Set goals, make a plan, and execute repeatedly. Don't let frustration of not seeing instant results get you down. You're working to be healthy and this takes time. While it's easy to activate bad genes, you have to renew yourself and get rid of the triggers for those genes over time. Approximately two years of healthy behavior will usually get things back on track. Most of the cells in your body turn over in that time. Essentially we become completely new people, healthier with good genes turned on and more resistant to those bad chemical actors from the outside.

Shedding Light on Fat Loss

Judy had tried everything for weight loss and nothing seemed to work. She heard me deliver a presentation on weight loss about identifying each person's triggers for fat gain and asked for help. Like many of us, she spent most of her day indoors at work, only seeing the sun briefly as she walked to and from her car or when she passed in front of a window. She was a highly trained technical professional and extremely successful at what she did, and yet her health had suffered. I admired her willingness to try something new and wanted to give her a quick and easy boost. I asked her to get outside in the sun for ten to fifteen minutes each day, in the morning, at noon, and just before sunset. This changed her life and outlook, and made her weight loss start and stay on track. She was excited when she showed me she could wear her wedding ring for the first time in years.

By using a simple trick, she reset her internal clock and told her body it was time to give up the body fat. She slept better, felt better, and had regular progress in weight loss and dropping sizes. There is a normal internal daily and seasonal clock in your body. These clocks give you the ability to react to daily and seasonal variation in environmental conditions. Multiple cells of your body are sensitive to environmental signals of time and season. This lets the cellular community work together to give the behavior and reactions most likely to lead to survival. But just like a real clock, your internal clock can be off or broken. When your internal and seasonal clocks are not synchronized to the world around you, bad things happen.

Seasonal Light

Sunlight is important to the functioning of your internal clock. It works in several different ways: direct impact on your skin, production of vitamin D, and detection by your hair follicles (Iyengar, 1998) and retinas. Each plays a role and works to varying degrees in different people. Obviously, someone who is blind will register less of an impact from the eyes. The key is to maximize methods of sunlight intake. Sunlight is an essential nutrient that when absent causes symptoms of deficiency. How do you prevent this deficiency and what is the natural timing to help you get back on track?

Normally, spring and summer has exposure to bright sunlight for more hours of the day. This resets your internal clock and seasonal clocks as well. Some people and races are particularly sensitive to seasonal changes and this results in normal seasonal shifts in their weight. This mimics the changes animals see seasonally. Animals detect the change in length of day by the presence or absence of light and the quality of light. By having a shorter light day, the fall cycle starts and animals adapt to prepare for the coming winter. As I researched the impact of day length on the risk of gaining weight, I discovered people are either Syrian or Siberian hamsters. No, I'm not calling everybody rodents. Your adaptation to the changes in light works similar to these animals.

Light response was shown to have remarkable differences in adaptation and explain the variations in obesity in people. Syrian and Siberian hamsters were studied to compare their adaptation to a shortened day length (Bartness, 1985). The researchers found dramatic changes occurred as each group was exposed to fall lighting conditions (shorter days). The Syrian group added fat weight to store up enough energy to survive the winter. This increased their fat to muscle ratio. The Siberian hamsters raised their fat to muscle ratios by lowering their overall energy with reducing muscle mass. These adaptations were related to the regional availability of nutrients or calories available to the rodents in their autumn habitats. In one area, food may be more plentiful and so it makes sense to add weight, where another area with less food made more sense to save energy.

People fall into the same two categories of either Syrian or Siberian. Those who gain lots of fat but have a relatively normal muscle mass and look overweight are similar to the Syrian hamster. Then there are the "skinny fat" people who look thin, but actually have a high percentage of body fat. When we look beyond human studies, we see examples in the animal world of what we experience. Fortunately for animals, they follow normal cycles and lose weight throughout the winter. Unfortunately, we don't. As much as some of us would like to hibernate on cold winter days, we don't get to.

A study in England showed the difference between light exposures in the summer versus the winter, and reviewed the health and psychological implications of this seasonal discrepancy (Thorne, 2009). In addition to the overall increase in light exposure, more blue wavelengths are available during the summer. Both the quality and quantity of light changes over time and this is a key to your emotional and physical sensations of the seasons. You see less light in winter and it is different in quality. Today, people spend more time indoors under artificial lighting more than ever before. Artificial lighting has a very different light spectrum than natural lighting despite efforts to create more natural spectrum lights. The intensity of artificial light falls far below what you see in winter, and the quality of light rarely mimics natural light.

Seasonal Affective Disorder

This decreased light has an impact on how you feel and gain weight. Seasonal affective disorder (SAD) affects people during the winter due to lack of sunlight exposure. They can develop symptoms of fatigue and significant depression, and crave carbohydrate-rich foods. SAD also makes you eat frequently through the day (Cizza, 2011). That's not all. SAD makes you more likely to be an emotional eater, meaning that at times of stress, anxiety, loneliness, or depression you will be more likely to eat those sweet or starchy foods (Kräuchi and Wirz-Justice, 1997). The treatment is sitting in front of a full spectrum light to mimic sunlight or getting natural sun exposure.

SAD happens in places with little sunlight in the winter like Alaska, Canada, and the northern United States. Other northern climates around the world share this concern and usually have ways to deal with it. Since we spend more time indoors than ever before, SAD is occurring farther south. The southern climates are associated with sunlight and it is less likely that people there think of SAD as the cause for depression, fatigue, or obesity. It's under-recognized by physicians and undertreated. People living in sunnier climates have not been in touch with this risk and it's likely they do not recognize the problem. They will have unexplained fatigue, lethargy, and sadness. Even when the weather is sunny and they are doing well in life, they have this constant nagging feeling. SAD is insidious and causes a host of problems. A friend moved to Montana from South Texas and described the depression that came with sitting at home in the dim light of winter. Only bright light, sunshine, and visits back home made it better.

With air conditioning, constant indoor work, perceived outdoor heat, and indoor entertainment we have locked ourselves away from the natural treatment for SAD. The sun is a rare treat or shock depending on how we expose ourselves to it. We alternate between pale and cold to hot and burned, rarely giving ourselves the opportunity to adjust to the natural treatment to what ails us.

Sun exposure and lighting affects our mood, and the preceding discussion provides important evidence for the contribution of sunlight to weight maintenance. We spend most of our time in artificially lit environments. This has a significant negative impact on your health beyond SAD. Artificial light does not follow the normal day and night cycle. It extends the day at the beginning and at the end. When you think of artificial light you usually think of light bulbs, but that's only one source. Consider the electronic devices you use on a regular basis. Can you use them with the lights turned off? If so, they are producing enough light to have an impact on your brain and metabolism.

Phototherapy can reverse the symptoms of SAD. You can affect the problem of circadian rhythm by eliminating excess artificial lighting in the evening. But this is only part of the solution. Replace artificial light with direct natural light as much as possible to avoid the problems related to SAD. Phototherapy requires thirty to forty-five minutes of daily exposure but even people who are successful with the treatment have a hard time maintaining it. Getting outside is a challenge and support is sometimes needed to stick with it (Roecklein, 2012). I recommend people in sunny climates get outside in the early morning, at noon, and before sunset for ten to fifteen minutes each time.

Vacation in the Sun

When you go on a tropical vacation, you come back glowing. People will comment on how good you look and how your skin looks great. This is often thought to be because you're more relaxed. When you travel, your diet and sleep habits change—particularly somewhere a little primitive. You eat more fruits and vegetables, and things that have been caught fresh or raised naturally. This has a great impact and the effects can be seen quickly, even in one to two weeks. You also get more sun exposure and your sleep corresponds to the natural day. This helps you reset your circadian clock and have a more efficient sleep. When you go to a place where you are up all night and sleep late, or continue on the same diet you don't get that same benefit.

Look at your pictures from Florida, Cancun, Costa Rica, or any other sunny or tropical place you may have visited. Remember the great fresh food and seafood you ate? You'll notice there was a lot of starch in the diet but very few were wheat based. You might have had tortillas or bread but likely you were eating other starches such as plantain, yucca, and beans. You may have travelled to France and had bread and other pastries in the morning. In fact, the French have a higher carbohydrate diet than you expect them to have and still maintain their weight. This is because the quantities they eat and the signals they give their bodies in fruits and vegetables help control weight gain. They are also outdoors and active a large portion of the day. Only recently with more processed foods and less outdoor activity and light exposure have we seen the start of weight gain in France.

The Hippocampus and Sunlight

Not only do you have a daily circadian rhythm but also a seasonal rhythm affected by light. The Syrian and Siberian hamsters are a good example. The changes stimulated by short day versus long day light exposure are remarkable. While hormonal and neurotransmitter changes occur, even more substantial and amazing things happen. There is a difference in the number of connections between the brain cells in a critical part of the brain called the hippocampus (Ikeno, 2014).

The hippocampus is responsible for differences in affect (how we express emotion) and emotional and cognitive behavior. Day length and sunlight exposure affects how the hippocampus is activated. More light equals better mood, better thinking, and better behavior. But it's not just the shape of the brain cells that changes. Light exposure will change which genes are expressed. Along with hormonal changes, you have changes in the shape of your brain and in how your genes are expressed when exposed to sunlight. Your environmental exposure has an impact on who you are and how you behave.

What else does sunlight do? Evidence shows that ultraviolet A (UVA) and ultraviolet B (UVB) radiation from sunlight has direct immunosuppressive effects. The radiation increases function of the regulatory T-cells in your immune system, and removes the T-cells that react to your body. When your immune cells react to your body, you have an autoimmune disorder, like lupus, fibromyalgia, Crohn's disease, and inflammatory bowel. Getting rid of the cells means less autoimmune disease. There is also good evidence that the overreaction of the immune system that causes asthma and other hyper-reactive diseases is related to sunlight deficiency (Kamran, 2015).

Other effects of sunlight include increased neurotransmitters such as Alpha melanocyte-stimulating hormone (alpha-MSH), Calcitonin gene-related peptide (CGRP), Neuropeptide substance P, and endorphins. How do these have an impact on weight? Alpha-MSH is an appetite suppressing neurotransmitter and when low contributes to increased food intake (Wilding, 2002). Other substances are also implicated in how we eat and are rewarded by your brain.

Your Circadian Clock

Artificial lighting and night activities have changed the circadian rhythm that controls every process in your body including rest, reproduction, metabolism, hunger, muscle building, learning, intelligence, and healing. It can be affected by fatigue, lighting, temperature, and stress—common factors of modern society. It's no wonder this generation is expected to live shorter than the one before.

Drinking water is important for your metabolism to run efficiently, and necessary for your circadian clock. Studies have shown water deprivation leads to interference with wake-sleep cycles (Martelli, 2012). Many people exist in a state of water deprivation or dehydration. Alcohol or caffeinated drinks cause water loss. What is your first drink of the day? Are you drinking beverages that contain sugar or eating more salt? Doing so throws off your circadian rhythm and affects your sleep. When the wake-sleep cycle is disrupted, less time is spent in rapid eye movement (REM) sleep, leading to fatigue and stress.

Artificial or Natural Light?

Experiments with people shut in rooms without access to outside light and cues resulted in them waking later, slowly shifting around the clock, and often depressed. We are locked in houses and buildings and darken windows to keep out natural light. Missing sunlight can cause health problems. Seek out natural light whenever possible to help restore your internal clock. In avoiding natural light, you are exposed to lots of artificial light. Not only are artificial colors, flavors, and sweeteners bad for you, artificial light is too.

Your circadian rhythm depends on exposure to light. Natural light affects your mood and weight, and sets your daily clock. Sensed by the eyes, sunlight directly affects the portion of your brain responsible for wakefulness. When awake, you are more active and less fatigued. When not fully awake, you feel fatigued and stressed. The shorter day in fall and winter-like lighting conditions that you experience indoors can stimulate you to eat poorly and eat more. Too little natural light can cause this, and so does too much artificial light. Extending daylight artificially causes the internal clock to go haywire. Light-at-night (LAN) is more common as we are dependent on artificial light and other electronic and light producing technologies. LAN is shown to increase depression, decrease connections between brain cells, and increase inflammation (Fonken, 2013).

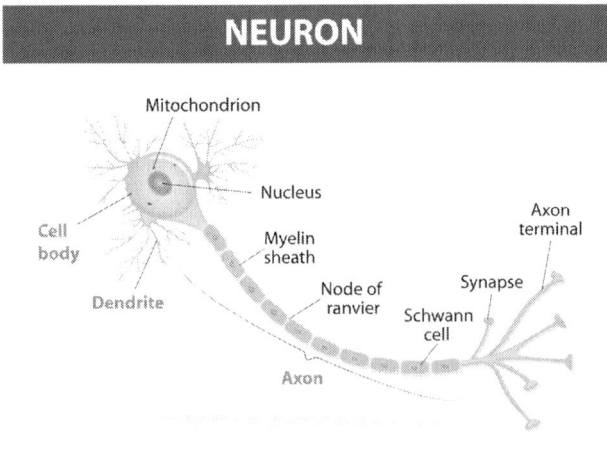

LAN decreases dendritic connections in neurons and increases TNF (tumor necrosis factor), a marker of inflammation.

Artificial lighting contributes to weight gain by abnormally prolonging day length. A study from the Netherlands (Coomans, 2013) demonstrates that prolonged exposure to light disrupts the normal circadian rhythm of an animal. Experimental animals were exposed to light all day or a prolonged period mimicking a long day. Their internal clock was disrupted, leading to an increase in their food intake by more than twenty-six percent. They also had a decreased energy expenditure of thirteen percent. The test animals ate more and had a slower metabolism. As expected, the animals showed greater weight gain than the high fat diet given to control animals.

Exposure to artificial lighting has a huge impact on your risk of weight gain and obesity. LAN increases your eating and weight, waist to hip ratio, waist to height ratio, and body mass index (BMI) (McFadden, 2014). This works out to doubling of the risk of obesity. No matter how you measure your health, your risk of weight gain is higher with LAN. The problem is more than exposure to extra light. LAN without sunlight has the combined effect of your internal clock being off, lack of vitamin D, and suppression of melatonin— your major sleep hormone. This contributes to increased obesity, cancer risk, poor rest and recovery, depression, and other effects on the body just being discovered.

The brain's central pacemaker, the suprachiasmatic nuclei (SCN), regulates higher food intake and lower energy expenditure. This part of the brain helps control your wake-sleep cycle. Clearly, timing of light exposure has a significant role in weight gain. Have you been sleeping later into the morning? Are your home lights left on in the evening? Make use of normal sunlight and let the evening be time for sleep and rest. When you pull out your laptop to read and answer emails at night, surf the web, or browse through social media for hours, you probably get more LAN than you know. The brain reward system has a big role with this, but so does the actual light from the device.

Melatonin, the sleep hormone, is produced in response to dark. When you replace the dark with artificial light, your sleep is less efficient, making you fatigued and stressed. Melatonin also increases leptin levels at night when insulin is around (like after a meal) to suppress hunger while you sleep. Leptin is one of the most important fat burning hormones. When you don't have darkness to stimulate melatonin, or fail to produce melatonin appropriately because of dietary deficiencies, you don't stimulate leptin in response to your evening meal. This makes you hungrier while sleeping. You are more likely to wake up and snack or wake up hungry in the morning, causing you to overeat.

Melatonin is also an important gut hormone. It controls movement of the gut and immunity. Anyone with gut inflammation or immune problems has melatonin deficiency as one of the factors. Weight issues can stem from absence of the materials to make this substance. The melatonin in your gut doesn't come from the brain. Its production in the gut isn't light sensitive like the brain melatonin that controls your wake-sleep cycle. This shows how many things in the body are interlinked and hormones play multiple roles.

A disturbed circadian rhythm puts you at risk for diabetes (Coomans, 2013), due to insulin resistance in the liver. The liver is where you store much of your extra sugar and eventually fat if you don't use them for energy. Insulin is one hormone that controls when glucose is produced by the liver. The ability to control glucose production is reduced by over seventy-five percent when the circadian rhythm is disturbed. Rethink that late movie, sitting in front of a computer, excess light in the house, or the night shift. Vitamin D is an independent risk factor for obesity from insulin resistance (Alemzadeh, 2008). Replenishing your vitamin D with regular sun exposure and supplements will help diminish this impact on the circadian clock.

Night Shift

Working a night shift immediately throws off the circadian rhythm. Artificial light of dim intensity throughout the work period, followed by bright light during the commute home, and trying to sleep in a partially lit room doesn't help. In fact, studies show performance during the night shift decreases when you are exposed to light reversal. Work, alertness, and performance are all affected when the circadian rhythm is unbalanced. This is important to know for employers who want the most out of the night shift, but if you're working at night you're at risk for weight gain, fatigue, injury, and illness due to this phenomenon.

This process can be counteracted by fully shifting the clock. Brighter lights that mimic sunlight during the night, dark sunglasses during the commute home, and sleeping in a completely darkened room will help (Crowley, 2003). Within a few days the fatigue, reliance on stimulants, and inefficiency start to improve. Adaptation can be achieved with little intervention. Imagine being able to impact safety, efficiency, alertness, productivity, health, and weight gain by making a few minor adjustments in how the workplace is set up and what you do. This problem occurs all the time with nurses and doctors in hospitals. The lights are turned down at night for patient comfort, which accentuates the problem for evening healthcare workers. Night shift workers often gain weight, have cravings, and snack more. Doctors, nurses, and anyone else are susceptible to this problem.

Are you getting light at night? Your laptop, cell phone, and tablet produce light. This has the same potential down side as obvious nighttime light sources. These devices also produce a different quality of light. The overall wavelength of artificial light differs from natural sources, such as sun, firelight, and candlelight. This triggers the disrupted circadian rhythm and can start weight gain. There are even worse problems associated with artificial LAN. Most LAN is in the blue light wavelength. Exposure to this is normal in the early morning and summer, and less so in the afternoon and winter. Having the wrong wavelength of light at the wrong time throws your internal clock out of whack.

LAN also causes a change in brain cell function. The genes for creating brain cell connections (dendrites) are regulated by the internal clock cycles. When disrupted, you turn off the genes for making connections between brain cells (Bedrosian, 2011). More connections between brain cells allow for creative problem solving, higher thought, and, most importantly, memory. Before LAN, people used to recite long poems from memory and recall events that happened years ago. With LAN, it's harder for you and your children to remember simple telephone numbers. Light exposure at night has a negative impact on the brain connections for creative thinking and problem solving. Laptops, cell phones, and tablets have benefits, but know the risks involved and make conscious choices to minimize them.

Light and the Internet

A recent Chinese study showed people with excessive Internet use had slower brain function and shrunken brains (Lin, 2015). The parts most affected involved decision-making and emotional control. Internet over-use and nighttime exposure to light makes your brain stop working, negatively affects your decision-making ability and emotional balance, and causes you to gain weight. Internet addiction is suspected to work by the same mechanisms as drug and alcohol addiction.

You're not immune, even if you don't play games that often. The app games on your cell phone have the same impact as other online gaming. Social media programs also act on the same parts of the brain. Frequent use of the Internet is a bad idea, particularly at night. Laptops, cell phones, and tablets should be shut off when the sun goes down. Put them away and keep your brain from shrinking and your decision-making ability intact.

Scientists use LAN in cancer research labs. Studying cancer poses several challenges. You can't inject cancer cells in people to see how the cells will act, or inject cancer cells into lab animals and hope they grow. A rat's immune system quickly kills the injected cells. They are foreign and have damaged DNA, and naturally eliminated by the rat's immune system. Research scientists shut down the immune system by exposing the rat to LAN. This causes stress and throws off the circadian rhythm, and allows the cancer cells to grow (Van Dycke et al., 2015).

Giving up LAN is hard. We have gotten so used to it. There are practicality issues in the decision to use light producing devices at night. I don't get much work done when my children are awake, so I need LAN to get things done later. The hour after they are in bed is when I pay bills online, write, read on my tablet, watch a movie or news story I missed, and catch up on email. Choosing to use the devices mean you must counteract the negative impact and minimize when not necessary. Once I learned about LAN, I shifted my device use toward daytime and keep it under tight control. By keeping LAN to a minimum, you avoid many of the negative consequences. Less than twenty minutes has little effect. Of course, if the twenty minutes happens three times an hour, you have a problem.

Growing evidence shows the changes due to circadian rhythm also disrupt the microbiome. Microbes play a role in obesity. Changes in gut bacteria contribute to many health problems related to obesity and poor health including nonalcoholic fatty liver, inflammatory bowel, and irritable bowel (Boursier, 2015; Sahay, 2015). Be cautious of anything that causes changes in the bacteria. If you have trouble with weight loss and additional light at night, your circadian rhythm is probably disturbed and gut bacteria may be part of the problem. Derangements in circadian rhythm alter the types of bacteria in the gut (Voigt, 2014) and this has an impact on weight gain or loss. These happen in as little as twelve weeks and have a huge impact on your health. How often do you turn lights on at night, watch TV, or use your smart phone or laptop? Each provides a light source when you should be enjoying the dim light of dusk and the darkness of night to help you sleep.

For Better Sleep

It is important to get adequate sleep, yet millions of people don't sleep enough or sleep well. Sleep hygiene describes what you should do around bedtime to fall asleep faster and have better sleep quality. Many things have an impact on sleep. The following is a brief list of things that have an impact on your sleep quality:

1. Light at night (LAN) exposure activates your brain to think it should be awake. Beginning at sunset, lights in the house should get dimmer until you are in complete darkness for sleep. Keep the laptops, cell phones, and tablets for daytime.
2. Watching TV preoccupies your brain and is a source for artificial light at night. It keeps you from sleeping efficiently. TV often has disturbing images, controversial issues, and other causes of stress.
3. Your house temperature when you go to bed is important. People sleep more efficiently at cooler temperatures compared to body temperature. Having a transition from warmer to cooler temperatures at night helps signal your body it's time for sleep. Be careful, there are a lot of myths promulgated by both fitness gurus and doctors about "ideal temperature for sleep" which are false. Cold temperatures in the sixties are actually detrimental to sleep efficiency in the majority of people.
4. Coffee, tea, energy drinks, and chocolate are stimulants. Don't take these within four to six hours of your normal bedtime.
5. Recent meals have an impact on how you sleep. Reflux related to meals or obesity may make it difficult to sleep.
6. Breathing is important. Sleep apnea and other breathing disturbances cause oxygen levels to drop and lead to poor quality sleep.
7. Daytime napping can interfere with the wake-sleep cycle and should be minimized.
8. While alcohol is known to speed the onset of sleep, it's disruptive in the second half as the body metabolizes the alcohol, causing arousal.
9. Nicotine is a stimulant and causes stimulation that interferes with your sleep.
10. Exercise promotes good sleep. Vigorous exercise should be taken in the morning or late afternoon. A relaxing exercise, like yoga, can be done before bed to help initiate a restful night's sleep.

11. Make sure you get enough sun exposure at the right times of the day to help set your internal clock. Older people should do this on a regular basis since they tend to go outside less than younger people. Three times a day—early morning/sunrise, mid-day, and sunset—is the most important.
12. Having an evening routine helps you unwind before going to bed.
13. Keep your bed for sleeping. If you expect TV, radio, tablet, or reading when you get in bed it will become a habit that keeps you from sleeping easily.
14. Meditation or prayer is useful to help the mind unwind and focus on positive aspects of life to take you into restful sleep.
15. Deep breathing with slow exhale will activate the parasympathetic nervous system (PNS) and shut off the production of the stress hormones.
16. Adding a good probiotic to your day can help restore some of the good bacteria that also have an impact on body function, including sleep.

Access to high fat foods all day will disrupt wake-sleep cycle and contribute to weight gain (Hatori, 2012). Too many calories from fat are like having a junk food buffet. A high fat diet eaten during a restricted part of the day (normal waking hours) has less of an impact on your waistline. When left unlimited you gain more weight even eating the same number of calories, and throw off your sleep-wake cycle with unexpected hunger and the need to eat again.

When you eat the same number of fat calories at night, you gain more weight and have worse sleep than if you ate the same amount earlier in the day. That is why people who count calories get frustrated when they take relatively few calories and yet gain weight. The time you take them matters a lot. Skipping breakfast and lunch, with having a late dinner is not a great way to lose weight. Eating fewer calories at dinner throws off your internal clock and will result in weight gain. Setting your meals (the nutrition you give your body) as a priority starting early in the day gives you the energy to keep going and prevent storage of extra fat, but you also don't want to skimp at the later meal.

This same result happens with any calorie-dense meal. Studies with fat, high-fructose, and high fat with sucrose yielded the same results (Hatori, 2012). Limit your food intake to the first eight to ten hours of each day when you see light and are most active. Following this schedule can stop or reverse diabetes and fatty liver, and lower cholesterol. Start eliminating risk factors from light and fatigue.

Temperature and Metabolism

An important seasonal change is the drop in temperature that tells you summer is over and fall is here. This signals many adaptations in your body. Some of them are helpful but many are less so in the modern world where we no longer have to struggle to stay warm. Just as important is what has been done to deal with heat. We have derailed this normal, natural signal and turned it into a problem. Challenge your perceptions of temperature. See if some of these good or bad adaptations are triggers in your struggle to maintain your health and weight.

The Myth of Fat-burning Weather

Everyone talks about the energy we need to generate to warm ourselves when it is cool. Ask anyone on the street, a doctor, scientist, or your mother. Each will say that you burn more energy when it is cold. Unfortunately, this is false. Cold has been proven an insignificant use of energy even when shivering. This idea is ingrained into our collective psyches from when we had to work hard to keep warm in winter with extreme cold temperatures and only an animal skin, piece of cloth, body fat, and activity stood between you and freezing to death. We rarely experience this anymore. In the coldest parts of the world people have modern clothing that keeps them warm even in subzero temperatures. But your body is able to tolerate and regulate a wide range of temperatures as proven by the people that lived from the equator to near the poles before modern clothing, heating, or housing.

As a youngster, my friends and I used to run around in the winter all the time. Our faces, hands, and feet felt the chill but we rarely shivered even in subzero temperatures. Running and throwing snowballs kept us warm and there was more danger from sweating and getting a chill than from the cold. Anyone who does outdoor activities in the winter (shoveling snow, skiing, or walking) knows the feeling of heat building in your coat as you exert yourself. But these are stories about common sense, experience-based examples. Let's look at the scientific research.

The changes in human society to deal with cold and heat have created the perfect breeding ground for obesity and weight gain. Although endurance exercise performance may decrease in heat, high-intensity sprint type activities and precision sport performance improves with increased heat (Mohr, 2012). This contradicts the idea that people perform better in cooler temperatures or in air-conditioned environments. Athletes who perform in high temperatures self-regulate low intensity activity to allow for the higher intensity burst needed in competitions without increasing core temperature significantly (Duffield, 2009). You were made for heat and can tolerate it well. Exercising in the cold when you are overweight results in as much as a ten percent increase in calorie intake (Crabtree, 2014). The cold makes you hungry, despite wearing clothes that keep you warm.

Have you heard about "fat-burning weather?" A friend who has had weight loss challenges for years told me about this. We were coming into work at the same time, and I was wearing a coat and she was in short-sleeves. I spent my childhood in Indiana and Connecticut, and young adulthood in Chicago and Montréal—I am no stranger to cold. When I asked if she was cold she said "Yes, but it's fat burning weather." I was shocked to see articles in magazines and newspapers on the subject shortly after. Almost as bad as the myths about fat and cholesterol that led to our health care crisis, is misinformation about temperature. Cold doesn't help weight loss, unless you are exposed to extreme cold, and doing heavy work or sitting completely still and shivering for long periods.

Exposure to heat (temperatures greater than or equal to eighty-eight degrees) results in decreased appetite and food intake. This is through increased ghrelin levels (one of the main satiety hormones) and decreased cholecystokinin (hunger hormone) levels. I was visiting Egypt for a week and we had an average temperature of over 110 degrees F (41 degrees C). Even with great food and family events, which I was sure would lead to eating more than usual, I found that our children weren't hungry even after running around. This was out of the ordinary. They are usually hungry all the time. Left to themselves, they would have eaten nothing and only drank water. My wife and I had to remember to eat, and not because we were extremely busy. Hunger disappears when it's hot.

There is also decreased weight gain with increased temperatures (Song, 2012). This may be due to the effect of heat on appetite or increasing day length.

Excess body weight can increase or decrease core body temperature, although this is not significant (Hoffmann, 2012; Landsberg, 2012). Even a modest increase in core body temperature over time can have a dramatic impact on energy usage in the body. If your core body temperature is steady because of excess body weight, you don't need to use as much energy to maintain your body temperature. Instead of being used for activity or keeping you warm, this extra energy might get stored instead.

Whether these changes in temperature cause the weight gain or are a product of the excess weight is not known. A decrease in temperature may result in lower energy usage for maintaining body temperature. It can have several different effects. Weight can actually increase with the same dietary intake, or you can maintain the same weight by eating less.

Dangers of the Air Conditioner

Another example of the relative ease with which we can heat ourselves compared to keeping cool has to do with the shift of populations. Initially, most people in the U.S. lived in the northern, cooler climes and were accustomed to harsh winters. This persisted for nearly two hundred years until a new invention changed our ability to cope with heat. With the introduction of the air conditioner in 1902 and its expansion into residential use in the 1920s, it became easier to live in warmer areas. Many Americans moved toward the southern climates. This allowed more productivity, as we were still a labor-based society. Over time, the balm became a crutch and an excuse not to venture outdoors.

Many arguments are against the idea that humans are seasonally weight-storing animals. First, we don't hibernate. Second, human fat does not generally make one more resistant to cold temperatures, like the fat in whale blubber or the dense fat found on hibernating animals. Third, most of our later evolution happened in the presence of clothing and fire. But you can't argue with the fact rural people in cold climates tend to be stockier while those in hotter climates are leaner.

People in warmer climates accepted higher temperatures, but now they see it is an inconvenience and intolerable. As they head outside, they feel the significant difference in temperature between inside and out. The difference between being in direct sun and shade can be as much as twenty-five degrees F (fourteen degrees C) but can be much higher with air conditioning. Anyone who lived before air conditioning played outside in the summer heat and humidity with no ill effects other than getting sweaty and needing a drink of water.

In the 1960s and 1970s when air conditioning was rare, children spent the entire summer outdoors, and adults worked in the garden—doing yard work or mending fences. Similar to hibernating animals, as spring came and the temperature warmed, and the green began to appear, people were drawn to the outdoors. They came out from their caves and walked into the sunlight. We spent more time outdoors with longer days. Today, we try to protect our children and ourselves from environmental extremes we tolerated quite well in the past.

Just like bears and squirrels stirring from dens and nests, we moved about. Somehow, even though we are now warmer in winter, we stay indoors. Even with access to plentiful clean water, shade, and the air conditioner if we get too hot, we stay indoors. Our artificial caves have a constant temperature and we refuse to leave them. Hiding in a cave used to be from fear of inclement weather and a predator or enemy. Today, it is normal to be indoors most of the time and record numbers of people are seeing the ill effects caused by the lack of sunlight in the form of various ailments including depression and obesity.

Turn off the air conditioning in the summer and tell your children it's broken. You might be surprised at what happens. I recommended to a friend she increase the temperature a couple of degrees in her house to help with her weight loss efforts and increase her children's activity. She turned it off, and was so excited to tell me what happened that she talked three times faster than normal and used her hands continually. The children played outside and jumped on the trampoline in the middle of summer, something that was extremely rare. She usually argued with them about turning off the TV and video games. She had tried to coax, convince, and threaten them to go outside and none of it worked. Making the indoors uncomfortable caused a dramatic shift in their attitudes and behavior. By keeping it off, she encouraged them to get out more, play more, and reduce their fat storage ... and saved on electricity. She actually saved money instead of spending it to lose weight and get her kids more active.

The air conditioner creates a higher temperature gradient from inside to outside. This creates a huge disincentive to be outdoors because your body detects change more than it cares about the absolute temperature. In the "frog in hot water" story, a slow increase in temperature causes the frog to boil to death, while he jumps out right away when he is put in hot water. While this is mostly false (the frog always jumps out), it makes the point that we detect sudden changes more than slight changes. The swing in temperature from indoors to outdoors can be as great as forty degrees F (twenty-two degrees C) by the use of air conditioning. That's not all. The average indoor air-conditioned humidity is much lower than outside. On an extremely hot, humid, southern summer day the perceived difference from inside air conditioning and outside can be more than one hundred degrees F (37.8 degrees C). How is this possible? Imagine having the air conditioning at a frosty sixty degrees F (15.6 degrees C) with twenty percent humidity and walking outside into one hundred and six degrees F (41.1 degrees C) and sixty percent relative humidity. No wonder you don't want to be outside: the temperature feels like it's over one hundred and sixty degrees F (71.1 degrees C) once you calculate the heat index.

Ever feel like you are going to die from heat in the middle of a city only to be surprised of how nice the same temperature feels in a park or the country? The inside-outside difference is a huge part of it, but city life is hotter as well. The average temperature is much higher in urban areas and can be reduced by adding or preserving green space. Plants reflect the heat during the day and keep the environment cooler, while concrete and asphalt retain and concentrate the heat in one area. Heat at night is lost more easily from the green space than the metal, concrete, and asphalt jungles we have built. As the temperature rises, so do the problems associated with it. Our efforts to escape the heat lead to more problems as we turn down the air conditioner temperature and spend energy on creating ice and chilling beverages.

Another very important side effect of air conditioner use, is where the heat goes that we take out of the inside air. No one considers this. Millions of structures with millions of acres of indoor space are air-conditioned. The first law of thermodynamics states that energy is neither created nor destroyed but merely transformed. The heat and extra moisture from inside air is poured back outside. Every day and night the air conditioner is running, extra heat and moisture are displaced from indoors to out. Is it hotter outside, more humid? You bet. This is true compared to inside, and areas where there is no human habitation. The perceived temperature difference between inside and outside your house is even greater than that heat index previously mentioned.

As a physician who takes care of infants, I see many families bring the children in bundled up when it is almost one hundred degrees F outside. They actually are taking very good care of their children. The children are kept in air-conditioned houses, transferred to air-conditioned cars, and come into an air-conditioned hospital. Their total exposure to the outside temperature lasts minutes, if not seconds, so the parents are protecting their children against the cold environment they are usually in. Makes you reconsider how cold you should keep the house, car, and places of business. If you are afraid your children will be too cold, maybe you should warm things up.

Cool temperatures have a season. Stable, year-round identical, artificially controlled temperature out of sync with seasonal daylight exposure is not normal. Feeling the right temperature at the right time of year and the right time of day is important.

Heat and Metabolism

Animal metabolism, including humans, increases with heat exposure (McCue, 2004). That means you use more energy and are more active in hotter times of the year. Why is this important? When you keep the temperature too low, you slow your metabolism. That's not all: heat is an appetite suppressant. Anyone who has worked in the heat of the day for long periods knows this. One study looked at the effects of temperature on feed intake in poultry (Cooper, 1998). Farmers don't want their animals to stop eating because that means less weight gain and less meat production, less money for the farmer and higher meat prices. What's interesting is you can use this information to benefit your health and weight loss. In that study, animals exposed to heat ate much less and gained weight much slower.

Animals living in desert climates are never fat. Rabbits and deer living in the Arizona desert are slim and small. While driving from Phoenix to the Grand Canyon, you'll see jackrabbits, deer, antelope, coyotes, and many bird species. They are slim and carry very little body fat. When you get to higher elevations and cooler climates closer to the Canyon, you see bigger animals such as elk and bear. These animals have more size but also average more body fat than animals from the hotter regions.

Deer in northern climates where it gets cold are very different from those in the south. White-tailed deer in Pennsylvania are nearly four times the size of those in south Texas. As an adopted Texan, I take pride in everything being bigger in Texas, but this is an exception. Free-range sheep, cows, and chickens exposed to the heat have very little fat. Compared to animals in colder climates they look downright anorexic. Farmers use this to their advantage by air-conditioning their barns to keep the animals cool and stimulate their appetites to keep them happily eating their way to higher weights.

Desert-dwellers are rarely overweight. Only when air conditioning and western diet are introduced will people in hot regions gain weight. India is a good example. Western diets and air-conditioning prompt more obesity in a region where it was once rare. Another example is the Middle East. Obesity grows in regions of affluence where people compete to show their wealth and success by adding western, processed fast food to the diet and air-conditioning to the home and work place. Obesity also occurs in areas of poverty where people are convinced it is cheaper to eat unhealthy than healthy. Yet, another example is the Philippines. Obesity was rare on this tropical island chain particularly since the preferred method of transportation was walking. While incidences of obesity are less than in the U.S., the islands have more today than ten years ago. People frequently replace what they believe to be expensive foods with cheaper alternatives completely forgetting that the "expensive foods" were the same their parents ate for pennies just years before. These were consumed in smaller quantities and led to fewer cravings since they contained more nutrition. Most of what are considered "expensive foods" are cheaper and can be grown in a home garden.

With sun exposure and constant heat in warmer parts of the world, your body gets what it needs to give up excess fat. Your body works harder to get rid of the heat, which uses more energy, and gives up the fat so it doesn't hold in more heat. Native people who live on subsistence farming and exposed to the ambient temperatures tend to be slimmer with few notable exceptions. Those adopting modern lifestyles and diets, and have excessive leisure time that goes unfilled with activity tend to attain body shapes very different from their ancestors.

Cold and Metabolism

In colder temperatures, you shiver. Shivering is muscle contraction and uses energy. Shouldn't that help offset weight gain? First, you don't shiver at normal air-conditioning temperatures unless you intentionally torture yourself with cold. Second, shivering burns about four hundred calories per hour, about the same as walking at 4.5 mph (that's a thirteen-minute mile if you're trying to time it). When you exercise, you generate excess heat you need to get rid of and shivering stops. You have to be still in the cold for the hour to lose four hundred calories. Anyone who has hiked in winter or shoveled snow knows how hot you can get. In fact, you have to be careful not to sweat to prevent rapid chilling after stopping the exercise. If staying in the cold and shivering for an hour sounds like fun, give it a try. Instead, let's see what happens in the cold and figure out how you can avoid the problems or take advantage of the opportunities.

An animal's metabolism slows down in the cold, and they go into torpor (prolonged sleep with slow metabolism) or hibernation when it gets cold enough. People have similar reactions to temperature. In the winter or cold weather, you don't want to get out from under the bedcovers. It's not just the temperature difference. There are physiologic reasons why you want to sleep more in the winter. The problem is even though your body prepares for winter similar to other animals you don't hibernate. You never lose the excess weight you packed on since you never stop eating to allow burning of the stored energy. Cold temperatures act as a stress to the body and cause an increase in cortisol and ghrelin. Both are appetite-stimulating hormones (Geliebter, 2013).

These changes in hormones affect your taste perception as well. You start to prefer sweeter foods. The cold-related cortisol increase causes your taste intensity perception to decrease (Al'Absi, 2012). That means you need more sugar in your coffee drink in the winter to give the same perception of sweet. Have you ever been to a warm coffee shop? Try this experiment: order your favorite hot coffee drink with all the sweeteners and sit outside in the hottest part of a summer day to drink it. If you can finish it, you are indeed amazing. Try that same drink indoors and suddenly it isn't as sickeningly sweet as under the heat of the sun. By adding ice, we activate this same system of taste-bud suppression. Iced coffee drinks allow for taking the same amounts of the addictive neurotoxin, sugar, even on the hottest days.

These effects of stress and cortisol on taste aren't limited to sweet only. Salty and MSG flavor perceptions are influenced as well. You want more salt on your food when it is cold. Why does this happen and why is this important? By altering your desire for salt, you drive up the sodium concentrations in your blood, which allows for better cold tolerance. Unfortunately, it has more than a few other effects on the body. In warmer weather, your serum sodium is diluted and you hang on to more water. This allows you to sweat and keep cool without losing excessive salt. When you keep your temperature artificially low, your body readjusts and you tolerate heat poorly. It is no wonder that more people pass out when exercising on hot days than in the cold. They simply are not physiologically prepared. They are chronically dehydrated and refrigerated.

The temperature you are in and the temperature of food or drink alters your perceptions. Try drinking a warm soda. Leave a bottle of cola in the car and take a swig with it warm. *Ugh!* Not too many people can pull this off because when it gets warm it tastes too sweet. You not only get a change in flavor perception but you also get pleasure from oral cold (as opposed to cold on your skin, which gives discomfort). Oral cooling will help stop thirst (Eccles, 2013). That means you can be chronically dehydrated by artificially turning off your thirst center with cold.

Cold and the Thyroid Hormone

Cold has a dramatic impact on your thyroid hormone levels, the master hormone for your metabolism. When you are hypothyroid, your metabolism slows down and you tend toward weight gain. A raised thyroid hormone gives your metabolism a boost and you lose weight. The effect of temperature on your thyroid hormone is important to know about. It's assumed that thyroid hormone secretion from the thyroid gland increases in the cold. This would have the effect of increasing your metabolism when it's cold to generate more heat. This concept is one hundred percent incorrect. Many studies show that thyroid hormone goes down at most cold temperatures.

Studies of Antarctic people document the hormone that stimulates the thyroid gland going up but thyroid hormone going down. This is due to getting rid of more thyroid hormone despite increased production (Reed, 1995). We do know people in Antarctica require more calories to maintain their body temperature, so only looking at hormones doesn't tell the whole story.

Obviously, temperatures in Antarctica are very cold. To use cold temperature as a means of losing weight by using up more energy to heat yourself, you have to be extremely cold. Even if you believe you might stimulate weight loss with cold temperatures, hold on there, cowgirl. Before you run outside in the cold weather wearing nothing but shorts and a T-shirt, consider what happens to thyroid hormone excretion when the temperature changes. How much of the thyroid hormone remains and how much does your body get rid of when the temperature gets cold? You need thyroid hormone to keep your metabolism functioning. Thyroid hormone is eliminated from your body in your urine or stool. Cold causes more of the thyroid hormone produced in your body to be excreted in your stool. You literally poop away your chances of losing weight when in colder temperatures (Hillier, 1968).

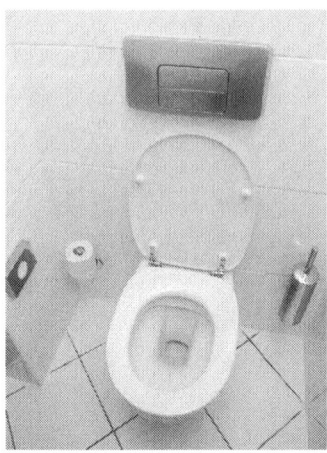

As much as fifteen percent more of your thyroid hormone is lost from the effects of cold. Still attached to the air conditioner? While a choice for temporary comfort, it is a major secret contributor to many causes for weight gain and obesity. Still think cold is fat burning weather? I hope you see that it is impractical if not counterproductive at most "cold" temperatures.

Another effect of cold stress is an increase in radical oxygen species (free radicals) that can result in DNA damage and even cell death (Neutelings, 2013). Imagine putting your body through this on a daily basis by sitting in air conditioning. While your internal cells don't get down to those temperatures because of your body's ability to warm itself, there is clearly a level of stress you are submitting yourself to. DNA damage can mean increased risk of cancer. How about getting used to temperature? You do acclimatize to lower temperatures, and the sensation and ability to tolerate colder temperatures will improve. However, this doesn't change how you get rid of thyroid hormone.

Cold and Health

The outer layer of your cells, the cell membrane, is made up of lipids or fats. This membrane gives the cells their shape. Without the membrane, the cell would fall apart. The membrane holds receptors that help detect changes in the environment and transmit those signals into the cell to make appropriate responses. The response may be to turn on or turn off a particular gene, or get the cell to move away from something harmful. These membrane fats are damaged in response to cold or alcohol (Marachev, 1992). The damage can make the membrane more rigid and more susceptible to damage, water loss, and aging. What happens to oil and other fats when they get cold? Animal fats congeal and some polyunsaturated "healthy" fats begin to solidify. This doesn't occur at body temperature but what actually happens is even worse. Cold increases visceral fat (the fat around your organs) deposits and not just in your belly, but also around your heart. You choke your heart with fat and increase the risk of diabetes, heart disease, and premature death by exposing yourself to chronic cold.

Chronic cold can also interfere with normal function of the receptors that keep the cell healthy and away from other damaging situations. This is important because the sensors also participate in the cell function. Cold sensors are even implicated as potential modulators of certain cancers, bladder function, and asthma (Knowlton, 2011). This means they may be responsible in stimulating cancer growth, causing asthma or making it worse, or making your bladder hyperactive. The next time you are sitting in a room cold enough to make your bladder act up, think about the other potential problems.

What happens to food intake with cold? You actually eat as much as twenty-four percent more calories and your taste preferences will be for carbohydrates. Animals lose weight in the winter by hibernating and not eating. Some don't move, while others are barely active. Do people do this? There are rare examples of times when people in a cold area were deprived of food and lost weight similar to hibernating animals. In a village in Pskov, Russia where food is scarce to a degree equivalent to chronic famine, people used to sleep for most of the winter in near hibernation (British Medical Journal, 2000). They were reported to sleep for five to six months of the year and get up occasionally for a snack, sip of water, or to put wood on the fire. Other rare examples of hibernation in people usually involve someone trapped in a blizzard or another freak accident in the winter. Normally you don't hibernate so you don't get to lose the weight like this. Knowing this shows you what to expect with the seasonal weight gain and cravings.

Cold also reduces thirst. You don't drink as much water and get dehydrated to be more cold resistant. Conversely, heat causes thirst and increases water intake. Cold induced dehydration causes increased sodium concentration. The blood becomes more viscous making the heart work harder to pump the blood. Dehydration also causes the peripheral blood vessels to contract to maintain blood pressure and bring blood out of the peripheral veins.

For those still wedded to the air conditioner and cold, here is a summary of the health risks I already listed:

1. Increased cortisol
2. Increased hunger hormone (ghrelin)
3. Increased visceral fat
4. Increased risk of cancer
5. Twenty-four percent increase in appetite
6. Thirteen percent decreased metabolism from loss of thyroid hormone
7. Dehydration and decreased thirst
8. High blood pressure
9. Thirty to forty percent less calories spent during exercise
10. Increased DNA damage and cancer risk

The Numbers

If you are a numbers person, you may have been doing addition while reading this chapter. Your calories increase twenty-four percent and your metabolism slows down thirteen percent. About thirty-seven percent more calories are stored, adding up to almost eight hundred more calories stored daily. This is with a baseline of decreased overall activity. When you continue the math to its natural conclusion, namely, how much fat do these calories turn into, a pound of fat has greater than 3500 calories. Imagine taking an extra eight hundred calories daily for most of the year. Say you eat healthy for part of the year and only consumed eight hundred extra calories two hundred days of the year. This equals 160,000 calories or forty-five pounds gained in one year. See how easy it is to pack on the pounds? Your natural response to temperature had nothing to do with overeating. These were biologically programmed responses. But even the most primitive biological imperatives can be counteracted or overcome with the right knowledge and tools. Change is possible, it just requires beginning and continuing.

Fixing Your Temperature Signals

After talking about the disasters that will befall you from air-conditioning, let's find out how we can fix the problem without resorting to running around the plains in a loin cloth. Many fitness professionals and doctors have the wrong perception about temperature. They believe being cool during exercise helps you perform better. While endurance sports may benefit from cooler temperatures, a great deal of scientific evidence shows that warmer temperatures improve athletic performance. Animals, including humans, did not originally develop in areas of cold temperatures. We came from a region that was relatively warm. All of your body's metabolic processes function at a relatively high temperature. In fact, the efficiency gained at slightly higher temperatures is lost when body temperature drops.

Another reason for recommending exercise at cooler temperatures is the belief it takes greater energy expenditure at cooler temperatures to keep the body warm than energy needed at warm temperatures to keep cool. This concept was laid to rest in the 1960s. Studies have been done to determine energy usage by the body to stay warm or cool. Most exercise in the U.S. is performed in air-conditioned facilities. The thermostats are set from temperate to cool, and far from the cold of winter. It is important to know what happens when the temperature is lower or goes up. What occurs to your calorie usage doing exercise under these conditions? The caloric need for the average male or female doing heavy exercise in moderate or air-conditioned temperatures is

3300 to 4100 calories per day. This refers to hours of hard physical activity throughout the day, not just thirty minutes to an hour spent in the gym. In extreme cold temperatures with significant exercise, energy requirements increase to 3600 to 4400 calories. This means an almost ten percent increase in extreme cold, much less than fifty degrees F. When was the last time you spent a day of hard labor outside in the middle of a freezing winter? Okay, you Great Lakes military folks don't count.

The cold temperature gain of ten percent energy usage seems a significant amount until you consider how much energy is used in high heat. It takes 4200 to 4800 calories to perform the same amount of work at one hundred degrees F (37.8 degrees C) (Consolazio, 1963). Six hundred to twelve hundred more calories are burned at higher rather than freezing temperatures, an almost thirty percent increase over exercising at moderate temperatures or in air-conditioning. Another study supported this finding of higher energy requirements in summer temperatures with significant physical activity (Burstein, 1996). The cold increases energy use only at extremely low winter temperatures, not the neutral temperatures of air-conditioning or fall, or when you try to skip the heat of summer and escape to the cool inside.

High temperatures cause increased caloric needs for many reasons. First, heart rate increases at higher temperatures above what the activity level requires to allow for heat dissipation. This uses a lot of energy. Second, metabolic activity naturally increases at higher temperatures because of improved efficiency in your enzyme function. Third, sweat contains protein and you lose more as you sweat. Your protein intake has to be increased and work is needed to digest the extra protein, and requires additional energy.

Any soldier who did a tour of duty in the Iraqi desert will tell you they had to eat like crazy to keep up their energy levels. Most describe being in the best shape of their lives, not just functionally but also in how slim and defined they were. The military knew this and fed the soldiers accordingly. No fat soldiers came back from the desert, but this wasn't just because they hiked and carried heavy packs. Regular activity in the heat of the desert helped raise their energy use. I don't suggest exercising in the desert, or working out during the hottest part of the day, but do some of your activity in the real temperatures of the environment.

Energy Usage

Metabolism in men and women is significantly different. The metabolic heat generated during the same level of exercise results in fifteen to twenty percent differences in energy output (Gagnon, 2008). This is another explanation why men can exercise and lose weight faster than women, and may be related to differences in muscle mass or the efficiency of energy use during exercise. Women should not be discouraged. The key is to use all these tricks, facts, and tools to your advantage. Real success comes from the planning, consistency, and awareness. All of the facts I share here are tools to find your weight gain triggers and avoid or turn them off.

Exercising in heat has a huge impact on energy usage, and acts as an appetite suppressant. Energy intake goes down after exercise in temperatures of 96.8 degrees F (thirty-six degrees C) or higher. You eat less when you have activity in high temperatures. This is due to an increase in Peptide YY (PYY), an appetite suppressant hormone (Shorten, 2009). Energy usage increases in summer to keep you cool by thirty to forty percent and your energy intake decreases. Get outside for exercise and you will reap huge benefits. Drink plenty of water and don't forget appropriate nutrition to build and maintain muscle.

My physical trainer moved to a new larger gym and had yet to install the air conditioner. When I told him about the benefits of exercise in the heat, he set up fans and kept the doors open to circulate air. The temperatures in the Texas heat were in the hundred-degree range. We got relief from being indoors in the shade but it was still hot. Initially, some people complained about the heat but over time, they saw accelerated results and developed tolerance to the temperatures. No one complained, even though the staff had to do a lot more mopping.

Sweating is the natural mechanism for cooling your body. It prevents elevation of your core temperature and allows normal body functions to continue. Sweating is fluid on the skin evaporating and taking heat from the body. This evaporation happens faster on dry days than humid, and increases with wind speed (Saunders, 2005). If you live in a relatively dry area or exercise in low humidity, you'll feel cooler and able to maintain a lower body temperature.

What is too much sweat? If the sweat drips off then you're not getting the full cooling benefit. Moving to where there is better airflow or shade makes sense. On the contrary, if you still produce sweat and it evaporates without leaving your skin dry, you're getting the most benefit. To support the sweating, make sure you're drinking adequate water. Electrolyte solutions are important for prolonged physical activity with high sweat production, but if you eat well and drink water you should be fine.

Temperature balance is not just dependent on air temperature and sweating. The food you eat greatly affects how your body maintains its temperature. The thermic effect of foods is how much heat a food produces when eaten and digested. Certain foods have a higher thermic effect. To maintain essential body processes, your body tightly controls temperature balance. The enzymatic processes involved in body functions are most active in certain temperature ranges and work less efficiently outside this range. Enzymes work in your digestion and hormone formation, building of proteins, and fat burning.

The hypothalamus is the part of the brain responsible for controlling our temperature and our food intake.

Thermogenic foods are those that generate more heat when eaten such as: hot peppers, black pepper, green tea, protein, coconut oil, and ginger. In general, most spices contribute to thermogenesis.

The amount of energy we store is less well controlled (Himms-Hage, 1989) than the amount of heat we generate and food we take in. Diet-induced and cold-induced thermogenesis (heat-making) are how we keep warm, other than movement. Insufficient thermogenic foods or inefficient thermogenesis from your brown adipose tissue can result in overeating, leading to weight gain. This is both a cause and effect of obesity. Brain control of temperature and food intake can be faulty in obesity, causing the problem and keeping it going.

Not only do thermogenic foods have a direct impact on the brain, but other food substances may act as neurotoxins. Taking those substances can have a great impact on how you behave and how your body uses energy. These toxins also act to interfere with the temperature control center of the brain. It is not just the thermogenic foods that contribute to weight loss but also the temperature and light of spring and summer. Since many people spend most of the day indoors, they never get the benefits from the environment.

Setting the Indoor Temperature

How cold should your air conditioner be set? The answer is simple on the surface but much harder to accomplish than you think. You must fix your temperature signals. First, adjust the temperature in your home to change. A static thermostat keeps the same temperature all day long. It makes no sense to have the temperature fixed in your indoor environment. Temperature outside goes up with sunrise and continues during daylight hours until late afternoon. At nighttime, temperatures go down. This is the normal daily cycle. A programmable thermostat allows you to adjust the temperature so you use the air conditioner only when you really need it. This eliminates wasted electricity (why keep the house cool when you are not there?), and reduces the huge difference in temperature between indoor and outdoor settings. This encourages you to be outdoors more often and gets your temperature signals synchronized to the day. Allow the temperature to get up to the eighties during the hotter days and bring it down to a comfortable sleeping temperature at night.

Second, allow your home to be warmer when it's warmer outside and cooler when outdoor temperatures drop. This seasonal variation in temperature gives you huge savings on your electric bills. For example, in South Texas it costs about $300 to keep a home cool in August (considered fairly efficient). By increasing daytime temperature when you are not home to eighty-five degrees F, dropping to eighty-two degrees F while there, and dropping the temperature to seventy-six degrees F at night—the cost drops to just over $180. A programmable thermostat cost $75. By wearing less clothing at home, using fewer bedcovers, and occasionally using a ceiling fan you can create a comfortable environment. A ceiling fan allows the air conditioner to be run four degrees F warmer while still having the same comfort.

How can you afford healthy food or supplements to improve your metabolism and help you lose weight? Buy a gym membership with the money you save on electric bills. Now, you might say, "There's no way I'm sleeping at seventy-six degrees F." As I mentioned in the chapter, "Shedding Light on Fat Loss," there are many doctors, fitness gurus, magazines, and TV programs that recommend temperatures in the sixties for better sleep. If you normally sleep better on cooler nights as part of the normal daily cycle, it's okay to turn down the nighttime temperature, get better sleep, and reduce your stress. This isn't the case for most people though. Why do you think businesses and offices keep temperatures so cold? It's not to make us comfortable at work, it helps the bottom line. It keeps us more alert. Research tells us a slightly different story than we were led to believe about what temperature is good for sleep and wakefulness. It turns out that 84.2-93.2 degrees F (29-34 C) seems to be the temperature at which most people sleep most efficiently. Above and below this we don't stay asleep as long (Haskell et al., 1981; Romejin et al., 2012).

You eat more, become less sensitive to salt and sugar, desire more carbohydrates, and experience a decrease in metabolism at colder temperatures. The overall effect can be as much as thirty percent more calories stored on your body or, up to twenty to sixty pounds per year of additional weight gain. Having something to counteract this on a daily and minute-by-minute basis is extremely important.

I noticed a few interesting side effects to keeping our house warmer during the summer. Our children drank more water and stopped requiring asthma medications. They were also willing to go outside to play in the heat and didn't want to come in. My family realized monetary savings and less weight gain, and more importantly, I saw my children regain a more normal childhood like I experienced when younger. That is priceless.

Fix your temperature signals by synchronizing with the seasons for weight loss. The cold seasons are usually weight gainers. Outside of a harsh winter exposure, spring and early summer are the seasons to lose weight. During spring, most animals lose fat as they run around searching for missed nutrients. By the end of spring, muscle starts to come back while fat gain is minimal. Muscle gain continues through summer and only in late summer and fall is the fat added back on. This is assuming you eat seasonally and locally and get outdoors more.

Brown Fat

If you live in a colder climate, take advantage of the cold although this is uncomfortable early on and can be risky to fingertips and toes if temperatures are too cold. Acclimatizing yourself at temperatures as low as the fifties will give you an advantage at that time of year. This means going out without a jacket and sleeping without a blanket. Some people have done this successfully, but it's not easy giving up comfort. How does this work? Brown adipose tissue (BAT), or "brown fat," is different from the white fat equated with obesity and poor health. This fat has the ability to generate extra heat during cold exposure without shivering. Research on BAT activation or increasing it to burn off white fat is still in its infancy. There are no definitive studies, systems, protocols, or claims this is effective in losing weight.

BAT increases non-shivering thermogenesis; your body warms itself without the muscle contractions of shivering to generate heat.

To achieve cold acclimation to fifty-nine to sixty-one degrees F (fifteen to sixteen degrees C), you have to spend six hours per day for ten days exposed to those temperatures without blankets or protective clothing. This will decrease or eliminate shivering while increasing BAT presence and activation to increase heat production by six to nine percent (van der Lans, 2013). Unfortunately, BAT is more common in leaner people and you can't predict who has or doesn't have significant amounts of BAT so this is not useful as a weight loss tool, yet it does have promise as a potential target. I mention this because many weight loss gurus have started claiming that you can boost weight loss by stimulating BAT. I want you to avoid this unproven, theoretical advantage that you have no way of predicting in yourself.

Using cold for weight loss requires prolonged periods of temperatures less than fifty degrees F. Either sit still and shiver or work out like crazy or take weeks to acclimate to the cold by not wearing a jacket or using a blanket. I don't see these as practical solutions for the majority of people so I don't advocate them. I have a better method that works in a much shorter time and gives great benefits.

A different method for energy loss due to lower temperatures is by swimming or exercising in water. Heat loss is thirty times faster in water than in air, and creates the opportunity to lose extra energy quickly. A one-hour workout will sap away a great deal of energy. The exposure to cold water also allows your body to learn how to regulate temperature better. Since the heat loss is dramatic in water, it doesn't take really cold water to get the same calorie losses as fifty to sixty degrees F air. You can do a workout in water and gain strength and endurance, increase your heart rate, and lose fat at the same time. Just as with any exercise, your appetite is stimulated and this may increase with the cool water exposure. It's not cold air from the air-conditioning or drinking cold water that helps, it's exercising in cool water.

Temperature Checklist

Correct your temperature signals and maximize fat loss by adopting the following:

1. Cooler indoor temperatures in winter
2. Warmer indoor temperatures in summer
3. Daily variation of indoor temperature with colder temperatures at night for better sleep and synchronization of the internal clock
4. Avoid foods that cold stimulates you to eat such as sugar, carbohydrates, and salt
5. Eat thermogenic foods that use more energy
6. Use swimming for significant calorie loss along with fitness gain
7. Exercise in heat when you can
8. Keep the temperature > = 76 degrees F during the warmer months

Air-conditioning has another negative effect: it allows more people to congregate in one place without being uncomfortably hot. While this seems like a boon to social interaction, it leads to greater viral and infectious transmissions. More stress, less energy expenditure, worse nutrition, and greater exposures to infection because of the cold is the worst-case scenario for weight gain.

Stress and Brain Rewards That Cause Fat Gain

Stress is important to any conversation about weight gain. A great deal of overlap occurs between stress response in the brain and how you perceive hunger and use energy (Sinha, 2013). Reward mechanisms in the brain and the hormones released in the body have multiple effects when you eat or undergo stress. A friend recently described his past addiction to food where he sat on the couch watching TV and finished a bag of chips without remembering he had picked it up. Stress, distraction, and addiction have a clear and complex interplay that is just beginning to be understood.

Many people worry about their jobs, whether they do their work well, and they worry about their children, aging parents, money, health, the economy, and politics. All of this has an impact on your wellbeing. There is also physical stress from strenuous work and play, injuries, and illness, which put a strain on the body. These have an impact on how you feel and risk further disease. The way you eat has a great impact and so does your activity. The light you are exposed to, environmental pollutants, and the sleep you get all affect your level of stress.

The ability to relax and get rid of unnecessary stress is important. Some stress is necessary. The only people who experience no stress are those who are dead. Otherwise, stress is a normal and necessary part of life. Exercise stresses the body but reduces overall daily stress by making your activities easier and releasing stress reducing substances as well as reducing stress hormones. Reading and learning cause stress in the short term but reduce overall stress by making you better prepared to deal with tough situations later. You can't sit on the beach doing yoga and nothing else. You have to live. By choosing what you eat, how you exercise, and how you handle life's challenges, you can reduce your overall stress.

Success can cause stress as well. Have you noticed how after a big success people are pulled to certain foods or eat out? This is similar to the hunt, after which the hunters ate large meals and more meat or farmers eating lots of bread after a bountiful harvest. They stored the rest of the meat and preserved it as with a harvest. The portions that couldn't be preserved were eaten first. They contained the most nutrition and helped the hunters recover from the hard effort they expended. When was the last time you ate organ meat or enjoyed a piece of fat? Mostly you tossed the bits that contained a great deal of the nutrients you need and counted on the less nutritious parts for sustenance. Your resilience and nutrition declines as a result. You no longer trudge on despite adversity. Instead, you focus on what could have been done differently, what could have changed, and what you might be missing.

The Zebra and the Lion

I was once shown a video by a friend marveling at the resilience of animals. A zebra was attacked by a lion. The zebra ran for its life and had a large bite taken from his hindquarters. He had claw marks and was bleeding but still managed to escape. The zebra, after the escape, did something extremely surprising. He did something no human would do. He simply put his head down and started grazing again. He didn't relive the experience over and over. He didn't question his decision to run versus fight. He didn't back track to his childhood when he could have learned how to better avoid the lion. He simply was done with that event and was living in the present moment. He could not change what had happened but he could change what was currently happening. If he stopped eating and became worried about lions he would die of starvation or he would weaken from not healing his wound. Living in the past would distract him from the future and he might not notice the next lion because he was so focused on the last one.

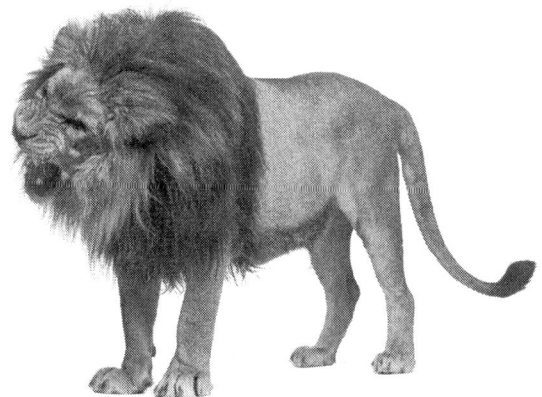

Every day you deal with lions, some of them real and many imaginary. You add stress to your life by adding excessive decisions that give you the illusion of freedom. Walk into a fast food restaurant and look at the menu to decide what you will have. You have that menu memorized, you know exactly what you order ninety-nine percent of the time, and yet you stand frozen by a decision that is simple. Everyone does this in one way or another. Which ice cream flavor to order, which cereal, what colored shirt are examples where this kind of repetitive decision-making happens. When the choices are limited to strawberry, vanilla, and chocolate, the decision is much easier because the contrast is so great that it's hard to regret not picking a flavor you like. The more choices you have, the worse decisions you tend to make (Vohs, 2008). Make those choice decisions ahead of time to avoid the stress. Decide the menu option when you only have what is in your imagination, and not the distracting hundred items you never order. This decision-making, or indecision-making, adds a lot of stress.

Excessive options add stress and you are likely to make poor choices. Studies show that too many options encourage people to eat twenty percent more than they would with fewer choices. Like hitting the buffet or Thanksgiving dinner, you see so much variety that you try several extra food types than normal. You eat more than you planned and should. Restaurants and fast food places know this simple psychology. They provide choices to satisfy more customers, and the benefit of twenty percent increased sales never hurts their bottom line. It does, however, hurt yours.

Many people feel guilty after a big meal when they eat more than they should, and stress from the guilt can cause greater weight gain than the excess calories. The stress hormones cortisol and epinephrine make your body store fat and eat more. This is why I teach my patients to be mindful in decision-making, as well as mindful in eating. Decide ahead of time what you really want and then carry it out rather than waiting until you are faced with too many choices. For example, choose the flavor of ice cream before you go out: "I'm going to have strawberry and if they don't have strawberry I'll have chocolate." Now, the decision is easy. You walk up to the counter relaxed and ready to order.

Try This at Home

When you have the desire to eat, think about what you really crave. Don't just open the cupboard and stare, or stand in front of an open refrigerator door going through possible items and combinations. Deciding first takes away a lot of stress and eliminates options you don't want to begin with. You already know what you have to eat in the house because you bought it and put it there. If it's been there long enough to forget, you might not want to eat it anyway.

This also helps cut back on unnecessary calories, because most of the excess calories you consume under stress originate from snacking. Energy drinks, cookies, or a handful of nuts goes a long way, especially when you continue the habit over time. According to research, seventy-three percent of people experience this increase in snacking with stress (Sinha, 2013; Oliver, 1999). When you succumb to stress-related snacking, it's not celery and kale salad you reach for. You usually pick calorie-dense foods such as fast foods and snacks. This is why it's important to keep track of what you eat in the beginning of your weight loss effort and when you meet challenges.

Your body doesn't care what causes the stress: it could be a lion or deciding what size of fries to have with your burger. Stress is stress and results in significant consequences. Imagined or real, the stress response is the same and can lead to fat gain (Jastreboff, 2013). Post-traumatic stress disorder (PTSD) is an extreme form that illustrates the point. People relive a traumatic moment and react physiologically. The zebra drops the stress, sheds the stress hormones, and goes back to normal activity. Other things cause milder reactions, but are still significant. This is because people confuse freedom with choice. More choice doesn't make you free. Principled action is more liberating than having to decide every time the "best" thing to do. Avoid PTBD (post traumatic burger disorder) and be clear on your plans and choices before you're in the situation that requires a decision.

Stress Response

The lack of sleep through prolonged work hours, daylight savings time, or poor sleep quality leads to significant fatigue and stress. Fatigue contributes to the problem of circadian rhythm by causing stress, adding hormones that contribute to weight gain. As a species, we have a well-developed fight or flight response that drives us to run and hide when we can't face or overcome fear. This was an important adaptation to avoid bad weather or defend against a large number of predators. Anyone who has driven above the speed limit and seen the flashing lights behind them knows the sensation of rapid heartbeat and tightness in the stomach that heralds the fight or flight response. Rarely is it activated for a real threat any more. Yet, we continue to hide indoors.

You have built-in instincts for many things and even though they may be dulled, they are still there. When you react as if you are afraid and hiding from something, what impact does that have on your stress response? Leaving the cave lets your fear level drop and resets your stress response. By staying indoors, even vague fears and unlikely events become a greater concern. The media convinces you of threats outdoors, dangers in the community, and risks of death to the unwary that stray from home.

Even without an immediate threat, anyone who has watched a political discussion knows how this can trigger the stress response. Yelling at the TV about a politician is the same fight or flight response. Since there is no immediate threat, the fight side is activated. You go to the movies for the same rush of hormones and emotion. Night after night, you treat your body to the same sensations as if a lion were chasing you, yet you can't escape. The lion keeps coming. It's no wonder you are tired. Imagine running from lions, tigers, and bears every day. Even your hearty caveman ancestors would have fallen over in fatigue. More likely, they would leave that horrible place for somewhere more peaceful. The friend who gave up the big city to go do mission work in a primitive place makes more sense now.

Flight or fight response signals come from hormones from your adrenal glands. Being chronically stressed increases those hormones and result in the body perceiving it's in danger. The perceived danger fuels the need for more food to supply the energy to escape from predators or a particular threat. When the threat is false, you don't spend the energy you intake for defense. This results in fat storage. Hunger helps curb your pain and fear response, particularly when you get hungry before being exposed to fear. Watching TV after dinner or going out for "dinner and a movie," combines feeding, stress, and fear, followed by sleep and a prolonged fast through the night. This is why you are tired in the morning, and sometimes wake to aches and pains, and a foggy brain. You've just combined the perfect way to gain weight. By increasing your stress with that movie right after that meal you will relive the stress more and will end up having a return of hunger sooner than you would have.

Maybe you avoid zombie movies and reality TV shows with people yelling at each other and sports, but I bet you do watch something. Watching the news causes an incredible amount of stress. Usually the reports are about what is wrong with the world. Essentially, it's all bad news, and women have a better memory for bad news than men (Marin, 2012). You may not be affected by one piece right now, but the next will make your reaction worse. That means a significantly increased stress response, and your memory for bad news actually improves with the more you hear. Thinking the world is going crazy or dangerous is a vicious cycle easy to fall into, and feeds stress and weight gain. Instead, you should be the zebra. The stress should only be there to help you overcome a life-threatening situation and then let it go, just like the zebra.

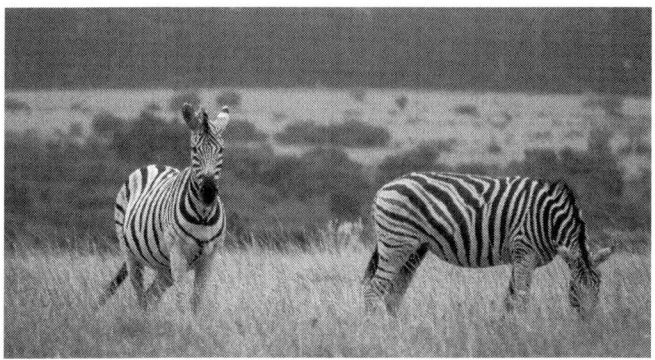

Stress Hormones

The body has two main stress hormone systems. The first involves the production of stress hormones such as cortisol, which helps regulate how sugar is released in response to stress. This is because sugar is quick and easy as an energy source. The second is the sympathetic nervous system (SNS) that releases epinephrine or adrenaline. Epinephrine shunts oxygen and energy to the areas you need to escape danger, namely your heart and muscles. It elevates the heart rate to increase blood flow to needed areas and makes respiratory rate faster. It also helps increase sugar in your bloodstream.

Chronic activation of cortisol or epinephrine heightens insulin resistance (Siddiqui, 2015) and can lead to diabetes, obesity, and other medical problems. Everything you are exposed to can cause stress. Watching a football game where your team is losing causes you to yell at the screen and curse a player, coach, or referee. Holding your breath at a key moment makes your heart rate and blood pressure go up a little. Later on, you review the game in your mind or talking with friends. This is stress, even if your team won, and the problem is that it's very harmful.

The same hardship and anxiety as someone playing professional sports happens to you, without the rewards of winning or the physical exertion. The body doesn't care whether you actually play football or tennis, and neither does your mind. People make multiple trips to the kitchen while watching sports. It's easy to consume a two-liter bottle of soda and a bag of chips, or stare into the cupboard for the next salty, crispy, sugar-coated snack food to feed the stress furnace stoked by cortisol and epinephrine. This is unconscious and often when you ask people if they are hungry during game time they will say no, but I need something salty or sweet.

You are programmed to take in certain nutrients at certain times to satisfy the demands on your body after a stressful event. Celebrations in the past served a purpose, the feast after winning a battle and the cookie after hours of shoveling snow was for survival. Not so much anymore. The components of life have been separated much like the components of food. Stress is taken out of physical activity and physical activity is separated from obtaining daily survival needs. A corn syrup sugar-high from celebrations nowadays give you a part of an experience and not necessarily the best part.

Another example you might think about is going to work, whether you like what you do and whom you work with. You might see something at work you want to fix but no one agrees on its importance or the people in charge ignore your suggestion. Other problems include meeting expectations or being disappointed by colleagues. You can work the job or the job works you. This is stress and if you are not equipped to address the problems, they will add to your weight. Long hours, short lunch breaks, and poor food choices are common in the workplace. More time is spent at work except for bed and the bathroom. Having these daily triggers for stress can lead to health problems. Money is one of the biggest concerns. You give up rest, relaxation, and evening eating time to get ahead financially. When you lose your health doing this, you have stress about getting it back.

Stress comes in many forms. A friend, family member, or doctor might talk to you about your weight and health, but is not sure what to say, so this makes you self-conscious. Even when you don't expect it, outside forces increase your stress. When there is no real stress in your life, you seek it out. Adrenaline or epinephrine is one of the main stress hormones from the adrenal glands. It increases your heart rate and breathing when scared. The feeling of butterflies in the stomach and rapid heartbeat when you see red and blue lights in your rearview mirror while speeding is adrenaline surging through your body.

People seek adrenaline from multiple sources. Some people climb mountains and others jump from planes to get their fix. How about watching an action or horror or suspense film that kept you on the edge of your seat? Your weekly TV show and the playoff games are sources of stress. They evoke an emotional response, which is why you watch. The TV networks bet on it. More important, so does the food industry. Snack food companies pay large amounts for advertising time during sports games. It's more than having a large captive audience. There is real psychology and physiology at work. When viewers have elevated stress hormone levels, they provide suggestions to cravings and taste preferences.

Understanding Stress

Everyone reacts to stress differently. When societies were less developed, people had different fears to contend with, like being eaten or attacked by a wild animal. We had real fears of starvation and searching for water. Most of us don't face these challenges any more. Many people in other parts of the world still do and their stress follows a more natural cycle of intensity and resolution.

Those who have to deal with these issues chronically also become susceptible to all kinds of diseases. Modern forms of stress about work, your boss, child rearing, and violence has the same effect on your body.

Understand stress and know what to do with it. Your body needs to be periodically relieved so you have a chance to recover. Relief of stress depends on rest, resolution of conflict, resources, right nutrition, and relaxation. One big problem with too much of the stress hormones epinephrine and cortisol is they direct your energy to the immediate needs to escape or fight. This means shutting down other body functions that are not essential at that moment. Chronic stress increases cholesterol oxidation (damage), tone of the blood vessels (higher blood pressure), and inflammation. Worse yet, heightened stress hormones shut down the parasympathetic nervous system.

The sympathetic nervous system creates adrenaline to deal with stress while the parasympathetic system (PNS) runs routine body functions like digestion, growth, reproduction, and immunity. The PNS is shut down temporarily to allow you to overcome the cause of stress first. When stress and fear are chronic, these processes are shut down to varying degrees over the long-term. This creates significant problems. Chronic stress interferes with your ability to deal with infection, leading to recurrent viral infections and the inability to heal minor bacterial infections. Women can have abnormal menstrual cycles and difficulty reproducing, and men can experience sexual dysfunction. Gastrointestinal disturbances such as irritable bowel, chronic abdominal pain, indigestion, and acid reflux are common.

Another effect of stress is on sexuality. It can reduce libido, and the number and quality of sexual encounters. This has a significant impact on self-image and potential for further weight gain. Sex is also a great stress reliever. Its reproductive function makes it part of the parasympathetic system. The PNS and the sympathetic stress system can't be active at the same time. Very few people think about the bills when they are sexually active. As soon as they come down from the euphoria, the temporary reprieve is gone. Sex is also great exercise requiring aerobic and strength components, and involves the high intensity interval activity that is so effective for weight loss. To get the best effect, maintenance and consistency are important, just like with nutrition and exercise.

You can have an impact on stress with simple daily interventions, and reduce some of the symptoms without medication, expensive therapy, or special foods. For example, consider praying before meals. Pause and take three deep breaths, and give thanks. Deep breathing with a longer exhale allows better functioning of the PNS. You can't run the sympathetic system with the PNS, and activating the PNS helps reduce stress hormones (Koopman, 2011). Dropping stress hormones before eating lowers fat storage and symptoms of gastrointestinal dysfunction. Omega-3 fish oil has been shown to also reduce some effects of stress (Carter, 2013). Not only does it have an impact on the risk of heart disease by reducing bad cholesterol, improving lipid profiles, and reducing heart rate response to stress but it also helps reduce the resting tone in your muscles and blood vessels caused by stress hormones. This means your heart, muscles, and blood vessels are more relaxed.

Try these simple stress reducers:

1. Make decisions ahead of time

2. Reduce the number of choices by visualizing what you desire rather than considering every choice available

3. Deep diaphragm breathing with slow exhale

4. Prayer and meditation

5. Omega-3 supplements

6. Have adequate, uninterrupted sleep

7. Address problems immediately, don't let them fester

8. Shut off stressful TV, radio, or movies

9. Have sex regularly with your partner

The SNS and PNS are only two of the hormonal systems that affect your brain chemistry and body in your efforts to be fit and lose fat. Several key brain neurotransmitters are responsible for how you feel and what you continue to do. Each of these has specific triggers and can help you on your path to health or hijack your brains to keep you overweight.

Neurotransmitters are substances that help brain cells communicate with each other. These neurotransmitter substances are dopamine, endorphins, seratonin, and oxytocin.

Some hormones have seasonal variation. Oxytocin, cortisol, dopamine, endorphins, and serotonin have seasonal variation. Your mood, appetite, reaction to stress and infection, and even pleasure reactions are affected by the season. Lighting, temperature, activity, and food availability modulate these substances. You gain the benefits when there's more light, warmer temperatures, and plentiful nutrition.

Neurotransmitters That Affect Your Brain and Waistline

The most significant neurotransmitter for obesity is dopamine, the addiction hormone. This was designed to help you stay alive. In the past, when food was scarce, if you waited until you were hungry you might not find food in time. To overcome this and keep you motivated, dopamine rewards you for identifying, getting closer to, and eating food. The problem is obvious when food becomes more plentiful, and certain types of food stimulate dopamine more than others. This same hormone is associated with many addictions, whether drugs (including tobacco), alcohol, or food. Dopamine produced the rewards associated with these substances. Our survival mechanism has turned into an addiction mechanism.

Endorphins are usually associated with exercise. These substances mimic opioids to reduce pain during exercise or activity. They act on the opioid receptors in the brain and reduce pain. Their purpose was to allow us to pursue your food and get a reward for pushing beyond your previous physical limits. Like dopamine, endorphins are extremely addictive. The same reward known as "runner's high" can come from sugar and carbohydrates. This effect can be very strong on some people.

In experiments, rats given cocaine stop eating and drinking, and even having sex. The reward is so great that it overpowers the normal mechanisms. When under stress, the response is greater (Blacktop, 2011). This continues until the rat dies, or you offer him an Oreo cookie. Then he will quit the cocaine and eat the cookie (Levy, 2013). They light up the same parts of the brain, and more than eighty percent of rats choose the cookie over cocaine. That's how they and you are wired. Food is very rewarding to your brain.

Obesity is triggered by seasonal signals, nutrition, and your own reward mechanisms. This disease is made of deficiencies, excesses, and addiction, and the amount is different in each person and family. Everyone who suffers from obesity has to identify his or her risk factors. The checklist at the end of the book will help you identify your personal factors affecting your genes and how much they contribute to your weight problem. The change of seasons synchronizes your internal clock. Your internal clock times the release of certain hormones in your body and what you do daily and seasonally.

Unfortunately, reward systems are hijacked regularly. Processed foods can be addictive. They act on the same parts of the brain as drugs, namely the dopamine and opiate receptors. Sugar is the most common substance that does this. In fact, sugar not only activates these receptors by giving pleasure and reducing pain, it increases ghrelin (hunger hormone) and decreases leptin (fullness hormone). Salt acts similarly, resulting in increased caloric consumption.

You also sabotage your reward systems when you go online. Social media sites provide a dopamine reward just for looking at the posts of other people. This is boosted when you get social approval or "likes." Spending time online takes you away from activities such as working, preparing meals, exercising, or spending time with the family. It sneaks up on you in ten to fifteen minute chunks that eat away your day. You continually reward your brain with happy neurotransmitters for wasting your day, failing to prioritize, and not doing anything to improve your health or relationships. It becomes an addiction.

Online Addiction

Take away a child or teen's laptop and they react with tears, emotional outbursts, and bad behavior. As an adult, you think you are more in control of your emotions. Unfortunately, you are susceptible to the same brain chemistry and your only advantage is your past positive, rewarding life experiences that compete with digitally generated rewards. People consider being online an escape, a way to relax, and in some ways, it is. The distraction keeps you from thinking about your life temporarily and provides a reward.

Here are a few of the signs that online use is hijacking your brain reward system:

1. Most of your conversations are about the latest game or app, or what you saw in a post
2. Eager to check your device for posts or messages
3. Involuntarily looking at your phone during conversations whenever an alert comes across
4. Irritation when someone asks you a question or asks you to do something when you are online

"So what? I get more rewards. I should be happier." The problem is this reward is like the participation ribbon at an elementary school field day, to keep children from feeling bad they didn't win or excel at anything. It takes away the motivation for real achievement by cushioning disappointment. Once you recognize this, you can start to limit your online time and make the rewards for positive activities that improve your health. When you reach a specific goal you have set for yourself, give yourself a big reward like a vacation, piece of jewelry, or new clothes, anything that is positive and won't negatively impact your health or the habits you are building.

18

Putting It All Together

Imagine for a second you are on a big island surrounded by shark-infested waters and looking for a treasure fifty miles away. You don't know where you are or where the treasure is. What is your chance of finding it and how long will it take? What if it's under-water or up in a tree? Having no idea where you are or location of the treasure are big problems.

Many people think weight loss is impossible. You can fix this by having clearly defined goals. My previous book, *Fast-Track Your Health,* provides instructions on setting goals, and a guide to devel-oping yours is available at **www.SpringCure.com/**. Also look for the videos posted on the website and Facebook. You're half way there. Where do you start?

Begin with your measurements: height, weight, waist, hip size, and fat percentage are important. Taking a picture of yourself is another way to see your starting point. You also need to find out what caused you to get where you are. It's important to know if the wind is in the wrong direction when you are sailing around the island. Learn the triggers that activate your fat gene and the solutions to shut it down.

Each trigger can have a huge impact on putting you into the fall weight-gain cycle. When combined, they can become an almost insurmountable force. Following is a review of the stimuli and corresponding solutions and actions to silence your fat gene. Go through the list and check those that apply. Now you have your own customized list of changes to make so you can lose weight, get healthy, and find that treasure.

Affects Me?	Trigger	Solution	Action(s) to Take
☐	Breakfast	Yes—quit; No—start	It's not the absolute that matters, it's changing your current habit. Low glycemic foods such as fruit in season and yogurt are an effective alternative.
☐	Carbohydrate craving	Replace missing vitamins and minerals	Take quality multivitamin with chromium, and vitamin D from supplements or sunlight.
☐	Coffee drinks	Eliminate	Decrease over time and avoid high glycemic or fatty items that go with coffee.
☐	Cold	Warm up	Set air conditioner no lower than seventy-six degrees in summer. Avoid ice-cold (particularly sweetened) drinks.
☐	Constipation	Increase dietary fiber	Take twenty-six grams per day and increase to thirty grams.
☐	Dehydration	Drink more water	Drink eight glasses a day or enough to keep urine clear and allow you to sweat with heat. Drink two glasses as soon as you wake up. The total should be based on one ounce for every two pounds of body weight. Use purified water and add berries, lemon and other citrus, cucumber, apple, and ginger to add flavor and nutrients.
☐	Deli meats	Eliminate or reduce	Replace with natural cold cuts without preservatives, additives, or flavorings.
☐	Dining out	Reduce	Make reservations, portion food before starting, and pay in cash.
☐	Eating late or at night	Eat earlier	Have meals during daylight hours. Avoid nighttime meals and skipping meals.

Affects Me?	Trigger	Solution	Action(s) to Take
☐	Emotional eating	Take emotional eating questionnaire (see Resources)	Get counseling, behavioral therapy, or coaching to redirect coping mechanisms.
☐	Food variety	Decrease	Limit the number of options at any one meal to reduce overeating. Change food types to achieve optimal nutrition all year.
☐	French fries	Eliminate	Stop French fries or add an extra vegetable when consumed.
☐	Inactivity	Increase with steps	Using a fitness tracker or pedometer, take over 10,000 steps per day to achieve weight loss and fitness. Increase to 13,000 if no results in two weeks.
☐	Instant oatmeal	Eliminate	Whole grain, slow cooked, and with your own flavorings will reduce sugar and glycemic index
☐	Lack of protein	Improve	Eat more protein or take a supplement. Optimum daily intake is one gram of protein for every two pounds of body weight.
☐	Light at night (LAN)	Eliminate	Sleep in the dark, turn down excessive light at night, and avoid light-producing technology.
☐	Monosodium glutamate (MSG)	Eliminate	Avoid foods with MSG, yeast extract, or hydrolyzed yeast on the label. Take a probiotic to help counteract.
☐	Not enough fruit	Increase	Eat at least two fruits per day, choose low glycemic when you can, eat in season, and only organic for thin-skinned fruits.
☐	Not enough vegetables	Increase	Eat in season and organic. Avoid genetically modified organisms (GMOs) and starchy vegetables such as potatoes, corn, and soybeans.

Affects Me?	Trigger	Solution	Action(s) to Take
☐	Omega-3 deficiency	Replace	Fish oil, seeds, nuts, and leafy green vegetables are natural sources of omega-3. Pregnant and reproductive age women need more to support brain development in future baby. Take a quality supplement.
☐	Poor strength/ muscle mass	Increase	Greater protein intake and muscle building. Commit to regular strength training exercise.
☐	Potato chips	Eliminate	Replace with healthy snacking, such as raw vegetables and nuts.
☐	Potatoes	Reduce	Choose colored varieties, limit to fall and winter months, and smaller servings.
☐	Processed foods	Eliminate	Eat raw, organic foods with minimal processing.
☐	Red meat	Reduce	Replace with white meat.
☐	Prolonged exercise	Work smarter not harder	Limit daily workout to one hour or less. Leave recovery days and plan exercise holidays, one week where you only walk, stretch, and jog lightly.
☐	Sleep problems	Make a routine for bedtime	Seven to eight hours is ideal but break it up if you have to. Avoid TV, light at night, reading, and stimulants. Take melatonin supplement if necessary. See your doctor if stress, fatigue, psychological disturbance, or hormonal imbalances are the causes.
☐	Snacks between meals	Reduce	Refined carbohydrates and sugar cause the formation of advanced glycation end-product (AGE). Eat berries and other raw fruits in season, and don't overcook meats.

Affects Me?	Trigger	Solution	Action(s) to Take
☐	Statin for high cholesterol	Eliminate	Appropriate weight reduction, nutrition, sunlight, and supplements.
☐	Stomach cramping	Restore gut balance	Eliminate toxins like MSG and take prebiotic and probiotic supplements. Eat live culture cheeses and yogurt.
☐	Stress	Reduce	Practice breathing techniques, prayer, vacation, listen to music, natural green space exposure, address your problems, get counseling, and add lemon to your water every morning and evening.
☐	Sweets	Eliminate	Stop eating foods containing high-fructose corn syrup (HFCS), refined carbohydrates, and sugar, and replace with raw fruits in season.
☐	Tobacco smoking	Eliminate	This causes a tremendous amount of damage to the body. Smoking cessation programs and medications are useful.
☐	Too much time indoors	Reset your internal clock	Get outside for fifteen minutes at early morning, noon, and sunset. Avoid light at night and get enough sleep.
☐	Vitamin B deficiency	Replace	Eat more green leafy vegetables, garlic and onions, and take a quality B vitamin supplement with betaine and choline.
☐	Vitamin D deficiency	Get out in the sun	Stay outside until you are slightly pink without burning to get enough vitamin D. Check your levels with your doctor and take a supplement.
☐	White rice	Eliminate	Substitute with brown, wild, black rice, and other whole grains.
☐	Zinc deficiency	Replace	Eat legumes, grains, nuts, and seeds, and take quality supplements.

Now that you've completed your checklist and understand what factors affect your body you have a better idea of what you can do. The key is to actually do it. Your effort must be organized and done gradually. It is unrealistic to expect to change every single risk factor for obesity and turn off your fat genes overnight. Attempting that will almost guarantee failure, like a person who has never swam, biked, or run trying to do an Olympic triathlon. You might survive, but you likely won't finish and may hurt yourself in the process.

First, identify your "why" for wanting to lose weight. If this doesn't make you have some emotional response it's not your real "why." My book, *Fast-Track Your Health*, can help with organization and planning. You can also find an exercise to define your "why" at **www.SpringCure.com/**. It's critical to have a variety of resources and a team to help and support you. Many people with great motivation, a lot of education, and significant financial resources will stall because they don't know where to start. That is why you're provided with a resource section at the end of this book. Visit these websites for more information, support, nutritional help, and find coaches in getting organized to silence your fat gene.

Weight loss and being healthy do not have to be done alone. It's not a sign of weakness to ask for help. In fact, it's a sign of great strength. Many people fail trying to do it on their own. This isn't a moral battle. No one says you have to conquer cancer or beat a heart attack alone. Trying to lose excess body fat is no different. Some things you must do for yourself such as identifying your "why" and setting your goals, but these are easy when you discuss them with someone who understands what you're trying to do. I have seen others frustrated by doing what they thought was good only to find out they wasted a month of effort. A simple phone call to a friend or teammate would have avoided the problem.

Decide which of your triggers to tackle first. When trying to get out of a bad situation, first realize you are in a hole and stop digging deeper. Pick the items that don't require a lot of planning. Setting the thermostat and turning off lights are easy. Add positive changes and increase to the more challenging items on your list.

Juggling is hard if you have never done it before, so start slowly. Add more when you are ready. Build gradually or you risk quitting your weight loss effort. Eventually, your new habits will be so well set they become automatic.

Small triggers are extremely powerful for activating weight gain, and equally powerful when you use them to silence your fat gene. The small investments in your health will compound over time. Albert Einstein is often credited for saying the most powerful force in the universe is compound interest. The same principle applies to health. Small investments and actions continued over time have dramatic results. Some changes will be significant and rapid, while others are slow and steady. Making a personal commitment to persevere makes the ride more enjoyable. Having a team to help you to your goal and keep you on track makes it even better.

Warnings for Weight Loss

A friend and mentor advised me to read books by Darren Hardy on business and entrepreneurship. Little did I know that the same principles I taught for weight loss, he used for business success. He described the same kinds of small, consistent actions in the *Compounding Effect* and described how they can substantially change your trajectory over time. Initially, the results may be undetectable but eventually they become transformative. In the *Entrepreneur Rollercoaster,* he warned about what people should expect so when they encountered hardship in business they could get beyond it. This seemed such a great idea that I had to add my own warnings for your weight loss efforts.

Warning #1: The excitement with any effort is greatest at the beginning before the hard work starts. This will dissipate unless you maintain it with consistent effort, learning, support, and affirmation. It will be greater still when you hit your goal.

Warning #2: Beware of praise. The reward from people telling you how great you are doing can motivate or sabotage you. This is especially true in the beginning when you haven't done anything yet. Telling others your goals is helpful if they keep you accountable in a positive way. Empty praise will not help. That "good job" and "awesome" may turn into sabotage.

Warning #3: Another friend and mentor reminded me of some great advice: put on your oxygen mask first before assisting anyone else. You can't lose weight if you devote all your time to taking care of others. Being healthy is a prerequisite for taking care of your children, spouse, parents, and work. Without taking care of yourself, you can't give your best effort and won't last long enough to help them into the future.

Warning #4: No matter how strong you start, there will be periods when you slow down in your progress and have doubts. This is normal. Having a strong "why" will keep you motivated when things get hard. Thinking about your "why" keeps you on track.

Warning #5: Look to others' success only for inspiration and small tools to help you. You are different and trying to copy someone else can lead to frustration.

Warning #6: Everything doesn't work for everyone. Though the fat gene triggers are scientifically supported, they are based on percentages and statistics from groups of people. Some people experience remarkable success for a given trigger, and others will have none or the opposite effect. Tracking your progress by keeping a journal, and having a support and accountability team can help you identify when this happens or when it's appropriate to adjust the combination of triggers and corresponding actions in your personal health plan.

Warning #7: Don't offer weight loss advice to anyone unless they ask. Not everyone is where you are right now, or ready to make a change in his or her life. Without knowing what they have already done and are currently doing, the advice may do more harm than good. Even worse, it may damage your relationship with them. Don't become the "food police" or the "weight-loss Nazi." People will avoid you. Only change yourself. Don't worry—people will follow when they see your success.

Warning #8: No matter how complete a list is for fat gene triggers, more will be identified tomorrow. I started with twenty and these grew while writing this book. For the latest version, see the resource section at **www.SpringCure.com/**. The current list is a starting point and you may find others specific to you and your family. Share any discoveries you make with the SpringCure team. You might see your suggestions on our website in the future.

Warning #9: Falling back to bad habits happens when things are difficult, or you experience tragedy, or simply get busy. Recognize when they get you off track and choose to continue building new, positive habits.

Warning #10: Don't be the hare! Going to the gym daily, working out long hours, and trying to make an overnight nutritional transformation won't work. Put in place the few things you can do for sure and add more over time to attain the healthy lifestyle you desire. This will avoid fatigue, injury, stress, and disappointment. Steady wins the race. If you are motivated take on a little more, don't base your success on your enthusiasm or mood. This varies and so will your efforts.

Warning #11: The majority of weight loss efforts fail because people try to go it alone. This is unnecessary, unwise, and definitely not advised. Build your own team and join our online SpringCure community, or online workshops and coaching (See Resources). This will give you regular feedback, accountability, and support for the success you want.

Realigning with nature, eating healthier, and making positive changes in your life can have a huge impact on your current and future health and weight loss. Use the Resource section to get help for eating locally, proper nutrition, supplements, coaching, and support. People fall into four categories when it comes to their health:

1. Those who don't recognize a risk to their health and don't want to know
2. Those who recognize a problem and don't know what to do
3. Those who recognize a risk, know what to do, and fail to act
4. Those who recognize risk, find the solutions, act, and continue to improve their health

I encourage you to be part of the fourth group. You have gained knowledge to initiate and maintain improvements. The only thing standing between you and success is your mind. Silence the doubts, old habits, skepticism, and the urge for a quick fix, and make permanent changes based on the triggers you identified as activating your fat gene. The actions you take today will be your legacy tomorrow. The SpringCure team is here to help you gain the tools and support to make the fat gene irrelevant. I challenge you to complete your trigger list, start applying it, join our health team, and take the necessary action to *Silence Your Fat Gene* forever.

References

Achten, J., and A.E. Jeukendrup. 2004. "Optimizing fat oxidation to exercise and diet," *Nutrition* 20(7–8):716–27.

Agrawal, R., and F. Gomez-Pinilla. 2012. "'Metabolic syndrome' in the brain: deficiency in omega-3 fatty acid exacerbates dysfunctions in insulin receptor signaling and cognition," *Journal of Physiology* 590(10):2485–99.

Aguirre, M., D.M. Jonkers, F.J. Troost, G. Roeselers, and K. Venema. 2014. "In vitro characterization of the impact of different substrates on metabolite production, energy extraction, and composition of gut microbiota from lean and obese subjects," *PLoS One* 9(11):e113864.

Al'Absi, M., M. Nakajima, S. Hooker, L. Wittmers, and T. Cragin. 2012. "Exposure to acute stress is associated with attenuated sweet taste," *Psychophysiology* 49(1):96–103.

Alemzadeh, R., J. Kichler, G. Babar, and M. Calhoun. 2008. "Hypovitaminosis D in obese children and adolescents: relationship with adiposity, insulin sensitivity, ethnicity, and season," *Metabolism* 57(2):183–91.

Antalis C.J., L.J. Stevens, M. Campbell, R. Pazdro, K. Ericson, and J.R. Burgess. 2006 "Omega-3 fatty acid status in attention-deficit/hyperactivity disorder," *Prostaglandins Leukot Essent Fatty Acids* 75(4-5):299-308.

Aranow, C. 2011. "Vitamin D and the immune system," *Journal of Investigative Medicine* 59(6):881–886.

Arsenescu, V., R.I. Arsenescu, V. King, H Swanson, and L.A. Cassis. 2008. "Polychlorinated biphenyl-77 induces adipocyte differentiation and proinflammatory adipokines and promotes obesity and atherosclerosis," *Environmental Health Perspectives* 116(6):761–8.

Assunção, M.L., H.S. Ferreira, A.F. dos Santos, C.R. Cabral Jr., and T.M. Florêncio. 2009. "Effects of dietary coconut oil on the biochemical and anthropometric profiles of women presenting abdominal obesity," *Lipids* 44(7):593–601.

Bahr, R., and O.M. Sejersted. 1991. "Effect of intensity of exercise on excess postexercise O2 consumption," *Metabolism* 40(8):836–41.

Banach, M., C. Serban, A. Sahebkar, D.P. Mikhailidis, S. Ursoniu, K.K. Ray, J. Rysz, P.P. Toth, P. Muntner, S. Mosteoru, H.M. García-García, G.K. Hovingh, J.J. Kastelein, P.W. Serruys, and Lipid and Blood Pressure Meta-analysis Collaboration (LBPMC) Group. 2015. "Impact of statin therapy on coronary plaque composition: a systematic review and meta-analysis of virtual histology intravascular ultrasound studies," *BMC Medicine* 13:229.

Baraona, E., and C.S. Lieber. 1979. "Effects of ethanol on lipid metabolism," *Journal of Lipid Research* 20(3):289–315.

Barrès, R., J. Yan, B. Egan, J.T. Treebak, M. Rasmussen, T. Fritz, K. Caidahl, A. Krook, D.J. O'Gorman, and J.R. Zierath. 2012. "Acute exercise remodels promoter methylation in human skeletal muscle," *Cell Metabolism* 15(3):405–11.

Bartness, T.J., and G.N. Wade. 1985. "Photoperiodic control of seasonal body weight cycles in hamsters," *Neuroscience Biobehavioral Reviews* 9(4):599–612.

Bazan, N.G., A.E. Musto, and E.J. Knott. 2011. "Endogenous signaling by omega-3 docosahexaenoic aced-derived mediators sustains homeostatic synaptic and circuitry integrity," *Molecular Neurobiology* 44(2):216–22.

Bedrosian, T.A., L.K. Fonken, J.C. Walton, A. Haim, and R.J. Nelson. 2011. "Dim light at night provokes depression-like behaviors and reduces CA1 dendritic spine density in female hamsters," *Psychoneuroendocrinology* 36(7):1062–6.

Belenchia, A.M., A.K. Tosh, L.S. Hillman, and C.A. Peterson. 2013. "Correcting vitamin D insufficiency improves insulin sensitivity in obese adolescents: a randomized controlled trial," *American Journal of Clinical Nutrition* 97(4):774–81.

Bell, P.G., M.P. McHugh, E. Stephenson, and G. Howatson. 2014. "The role of cherries in exercise and health," *Scandinavian Journal of Medicine and Science in Sports* 24(3):477–90.

Benton, D. 2011. "Dehydration influences mood and cognition: a plausible hypothesis?" *Nutrients* 3(5) 555-73.

Bischofberger, T., S.K. Cha, R. Schmitt, B. König, and W. Schmidt-Lorenz. 1990. "The bacterial flora of non-carbonated, natural mineral water from the springs to reservoir and glass and plastic bottles," *International Journal of Food Microbiology* 11(1):51–71.

Bjerg, A.T., M. Kristensen, C. Ritz, J.J. Holst, C. Rasmussen, T.D. Leser, A. Wellejus, and A. Astrup. 2014. "Lactobacillus paracasei subsp paracasei L. casei W8 suppresses energy intake acutely," *Appetite* 82:111–8.

Bjursell, M.A., X. Xu, T. Admyre, G. Böttcher, S. Lundin, R. Nilsson, V.M. Stone, N.G. Morgan, Y.Y. Lam, L.H. Storlien, D. Lindén, D.M. Smith, M. Bohlooly-Y, and J. Oscarsson. 2014. "The beneficial effects of n-3 polyunsaturated fatty acids on diet induced obesity and impaired glucose control do not require Gpr120," *PLoS One* 9(12):e114942.

Blacktop, J.M., C. Seubert, D.A. Baker, N. Ferda, G. Lee, E.N. Graf, and J.R. Mantsch. 2011. "Augmented cocaine seeking in response to stress or CRF delivered into the ventral tegmental area following long-access self-administration is mediated by CRF receptor type 1 but not CRF receptor type 2," *Journal of Neuroscience* 31(31):11396–403.

Blundell, J.E., R. J. Stubbs, D.A. Hughes, S. Whybrow, and N.A. King. 2003. "Cross talk between physical activity and appetite control: does physical activity stimulate appetite?" *Proceedings of the Nutrition Society* 62(3):651–61.

Boursier, J., and A.M. Diehl. 2015. "Implication of gut microbiota in nonalcoholic fatty liver disease," *PLoS Pathogens* 11(1):e1004559.

British Medical Journal. 2000. "Human hibernation," *British Medical Journal* 320(7244):1245A.

Brooks, K., and J. Carter. 2013. "Overtraining, exercise, and adrenal insufficiency," *Journal of Novel Physiotherapies* 3(125). pii:11717.

Brunstrom, J.M., and A.W. Macrae. 1997. "Effects of temperature and volume on measures of mouth dryness, thirst, and stomach fullness on males and females," *Appetite* 29(1):31–42.

Burstein R., A.W. Coward, W.E. Askew, K. Carmel, C. Irving, O. Shpilberg, D. Moran, A Pikarsky, G. Ginot, M. Sawyer, R. Golan, and Y. Epstein. 1996. "Energy expenditure variations in soldiers performing military activities under cold and hot climate conditions," *Military Medicine* 161(12):750–4.

Cani, P.D., and A. Everard. 2015. "Keeping gut lining at bay: impact of emulsifiers," *Trends in Endocrinology and Metabolism* 26(6):273–4.

Carmody, R.N., G.S. Weintraub, R.W. Wrangham. 2011. "Energetic consequences of thermal and nonthermal food processing," *Proceedings of the National Academy of Sciences of the United States of America* 108(48):19199-203.

Carter, J.R., C.E. Schwartz, H. Yang, and M.J. Joyner. 2013. "Fish oil and neurovascular reactivity to mental stress in humans," *American Journal of Physiology. Regulatory, Integrative, and Comparative Physiology* 304(7):R523–30.

Cizza, G., M. Requena, G. Galli, and L. de Jonge. 2011. "Chronic sleep deprivation and seasonality: implications for the obesity epidemic," *Journal of Endocrinology Investigation* 34(10):793–800.

Clegg, M.E., M. Golsorkhi, and C.J. Henry. 2013. "Combined medium-chain triglyceride and chilli feeding increases diet-induced thermogenesis in normal-weight humans," *European Journal of Nutrition* 52(6):1579–85.

Consolazio, C.F., R.A. Nelson, L.O. Matoush, R.S. Harding, and J.E. Canham. 1963. "Nitrogen excretion in sweat and its relation to nitrogen balance requirements," *Journal of Nutrition* 79:399–406.

Coomans, C.P., S.A. van den Berg, E.A. Lucassen, T. Houben, A.C. Pronk, R.D. van der Spek, A. Kalsbeek, N.R. Biermasz, K. Willems van Dijk, J.A. Romjin, and J.H. Meijer. 2013. "The suprachiasmatic nucleus controls circadian energy metabolism and hepatic insulin sensitivity," *Diabetes* 62(4):1102–8.

Coomans, C.P., S.A. van den Berg, T. Houben, J.B. van Klinken, R. van den Berg, A.C. Pronk, L.M. Havekes, J.A. Romjin, K.W. van Dijk, N.R. Biermasz, and J.H. Meijer. 2013. "Detrimental effects of constant light exposure and high-fat diet on circadian energy metabolism and insulin sensitivity," *Federation of American Societies for Experimental Biology Journal* 27(4): 1721–32.

Cooper, M.A., and K.W. Washburn. 1998. "The relationships of body temperature to weight gain, feed consumption, and feed utilization in broilers under heat stress," *Poultry Science* 77(2):237–42.

Crabtree, D.R., and A.K. Blannin. 2015. "Effects of exercise in the cold on Ghrelin, PYY, and food intake in overweight adults," *Medicine & Science in Sports & Exercise* 47(1):49–57.

Crowley, S.J., C. Lee, C.Y. Tseng, L.F. Fogg, and C.I. Eastman. 2003. "Combinations of bright light, scheduled dark, sunglasses, and melatonin to facilitate circadian entrainment to night shift work," *Journal of Biological Rhythms* 18(6):513–23.

Cunningham, S.A., M.R. Kramer, and K.M. Narayan. 2014. "Incidence of childhood obesity in the United States," *New England Journal of Medicine* 370(5):403–11.

Daley, C.A., A. Abbott, P.S. Doyle, G.A. Nader, and S. Larson. 2010. "A review of fatty acid profiles and antioxidant content in grass-fed and grain-fed beef," *Nutrition Journal* (9):10.

Davis, D.R. 2009. "Declining fruit and vegetable nutrient composition: what is the evidence?," *HortScience* 44(1): 15-9.

Davis, D.R., M.D. Epp, and H.D. Riordan. 2004. "Changes in USDA food composition data for 43 garden crops, 1950 to 1999," *Journal of the American College of Nutrition* 23(6):669–82.

De Vet, E., R.M. Nelissen, M. Zeelenberg, and D.T. De Ridder. 2013. "Ain't no mountain high enough? Setting high weight loss goals predict effort and short-term weight loss," *Journal of Health Psychology* 18(5):638–47.

Dhurandhar, N.V., D. Bailey, and D. Thomas. 2015. "Interaction of obesity and infections," *Obesity Reviews* 16(12):1017–29.

Dolinoy, D.C., D. Huang, and R.L. Jirtle. 2007. "Maternal nutrient supplementation counteracts bisphenol-A-induced DNA hypomethylation in early development," *Proceedings of the National Academy of Sciences of the United States of America* 104(32):13056–61.

Donat-Vargas, C., A. Gea, C. Sayon-Orea, S. Carlos, M.A. Martinez-Gonzalez, and M. Bes-Rastrollo. 2014. "Association between dietary intakes of PCBs and the risk of obesity: the SUN project," *Journal of Epidemiology and Community Health* 68(9):834–41.

Dubnov-Raz, G., N.W. Constantini, H. Yariv, S. Nice, and N. Shapira. 2011. "Influence of water drinking on resting energy expenditure in overweight children," *International Journal of Obesity* (London) 35(10):1295–300.

Duffield, R., A.J. Coutts, and J. Quinn. 2009. "Core temperature responses and match running performance during intermittent-sprint exercise competition in warm conditions," *Journal of Strength & Conditioning Research* 23(4):1238–44.

Dunstan, D.W., B. Howard, G.N. Healy, and N. Owen. 2012. "Too much sitting—a health hazard," *Diabetes Research and Clinical Practice* 97(3):368–76.

Eccles, R., L. Du-Plessis, Y. Dommels, and J.E. Wilkinson. 2013. "Cold pleasure. Why we like ice drinks, ice-lollies, and ice cream," *Appetite* 71:357–60.

Fabian C.J., B.F. Kimler, and S.D. Hursting. 2015. "Omega-3 fatty acids for breast cancer prevention and survivorship," *Breast Cancer Research* 17(1):62.

Ferolla, S.M., T.C. Ferrari, M.L. Lima, T.O. Reis, W.C. Tavares Jr., O.F. Couto, P.V. Vidigal, M.A. Fausto, and C.A. Couto. 2013. "Dietary patterns in Brazilian patients with nonalcoholic fatty liver disease: a cross-sectional study," *Clinics* (Sao Paulo) 68(1):11–7.

Finkelstein, E.A., O.A. Khavjou, H. Thompson, J.G. Trogdon, L. Pan, B. Sherry, and W. Dietz. 2012. "Obesity and severe obesity forecasts through 2030," *American Journal of Preventative Medicine* 42(6):563–70.

Fonken, L.K., and R.J. Nelson. 2013. "Dim light at night increases depressive-like responses in male C3H/HeNHsd mice," *Behavioral Brain Research* 243:74–8.

Ford, E.S., and W.H. Dietz. 2013. "Trends in energy intake among adults in the United States: findings from NHANES," *The American Journal of Clinical Nutrition* 97(4):848-53.

Gagnon, D., L.E. Dorman, O. Jay, S. Hardcastle, and G.P. Kenny. 2008. "Core temperature differences between males and females during intermittent exercise: physical considerations," *European Journal of Applied Physiology* 105(3):453–61.

Geliebter, A., S. Carnell, and M.E. Gluck. 2013. "Cortisol and ghrelin concentrations following a cold pressor stress test in overweight individuals with and without night eating," *International Journal of Obesity* 37(8):1104–8.

González, C., C. Gutiérrez, and T. Grande. 1987. "Bacterial flora in bottled uncarbonated mineral drinking water," *Canadian Journal of Microbiology* 33(12):1120–5.

Granfeldt Y., A.C. Eliasson, and I. Björck. 2000. "An examination of the possibility of lowering the glycemic index of oat and barley flakes by minimal processing," *Journal of Nutrition* 130(9):2207-14.

Guenther, P.M., K.W. Dodd, J. Reedy, and S.M. Krebs-Smith. 2006. "Most Americans eat much less than recommended amounts of fruits and vegetables," *Journal of the American Dietetic Association* 106(9):131–9.

Han, Y.M., J.M. Park, M. Jeong, J.H. Yoo, W.H. Kim, S.P. Shin, W.J. Ko, and K.B. Hahm. 2015. "Dietary, non-microbial intervention to prevent Helicobacter pylori-associated gastric diseases," *Annals of Translational Medicine* 3(9):122.

Haskell E.H., J.W. Palca, J.M. Walker, R.J. Berger, and H.C. Heller. 1981. "The effects of high and low ambient temperatures on human sleep stages," *Electroencephalography and Clinical Neurophysiology* 51(5):494-501.

Hatori, M., C. Vollmers, A. Zarrinpar, L. DiTacchio, E.A. Bushong, S. Gill, M. Leblanc, A. Chaix, M. Joens, J.A. Fitzpatrick, M.H. Ellisman, and S. Panda. 2012. "Time-restricted feeding without reducing caloric intake prevents metabolic diseases in mice fed a high-fat diet," *Cell Metabolism* 15(6):848–60.

Hector, A.J., M.C. Marcotte, T.A. Churchward-Venne, C.H. Murphy, L. Breen, M. von Allmen, S.K. Baker, and S.M. Phillips. 2015. "Whey protein supplementation preserves postprandial myofibrillar protein synthesis during short-term energy restriction in overweight and obese adults," *Journal of Nutrition* 145(2):246–52.

Heilbronn, L.K., M. Noakes, and P.M. Clifton. 2002. "The effect of high- and low-glycemic index energy restricted diets on plasma lipid and glucose profiles in type 2 diabetic subjects with varying glycemic control," *Journal of the American College of Nutrition* 21(2):120–7.

Henriksen, E.J. 2007. "Improvement of insulin sensitivity by antagonism of the renin-angiotensin system," *American Journal of Physiology. Regulatory, Integrative, and Comparative Physiology* 293(3):R974–80.

Henson J., M.J. Davies, D.H. Bodicoat, C.L. Edwardson, J.M. Gill, D.J. Stensel, K. Tolfrey, D.W. Dunstan, K. Khunti, and T. Yates. 2016. "Breaking up prolonged sitting with standing or walking attenuates the postprandial metabolic response in postmenopausal women: a randomized acute study," *Diabetes Care* 39(1):130-8.

Hillier, A.P. 1968. "The biliary-faecal excretion of thyroxine during cold exposure in the rat," *Journal of Physiology* 197(1):123–34.

Himms-Hagen, J. 1989. "Role of thermogenesis in the regulation of energy balance in relation to obesity," *Canadian Journal of Physiology and Pharmacology* 67(4):394–401.

Hoffmann, M.E., S.M. Rodriguez, D.M. Zeiss, K.N. Wachsberg, R.F. Kushner, L. Landsberg, and R.A. Linsenmeier. 2012. "24-h core temperature in obese and lean men and women," *Obesity* (Silver Spring) 20(8):1585–90.

Homan, M., and R. Orel. 2015. "Are probiotics useful in Helicobacter pylori eradication?" *World Journal of Gastroenterology* 21(37):10644–53.

Honma, K., S. Honma, M. Kohsaka, and N. Fukuda. 1992. "Seasonal variation in the human circadian rhythm: dissociation between sleep and temperature rhythm," *American Journal of Physiology* 262(5 pt 2):R885–91.

Hu, F.B., and V.S. Malik. 2010. "Sugar-sweetened beverages and risk of obesity and type 2 diabetes: epidemiological evidence," *Physiology and Behavior* 100(1):47–54.

Ikeno, T., Z.M. Weil, and R.J. Nelson. 2014. "Dim light at night disrupts the short-day response in Siberian hamsters," *General and Comparative Endocrinology* 197:56–64.

Ileri-Gurel, E., B. Pehlivanoglu, and M. Dogan. 2013. "Effect of acute stress on taste perception: in relation with baseline anxiety level and body weight, *Chemical Senses* 38(1):27–34.

Inoue, A., N. Yamamoto, Y. Morisawa, T. Uchimoto, M. Yukioka, and S. Morisawa. 1989. "Unesterified long-chain fatty acids inhibit thyroid hormone binding to the nuclear receptor. Solubilized receptor and the receptor in cultured cells," *European Journal of Biochemistry* 183(3):565–72.

Itariu, B.K., M. Zeyda, L. Leitner, R. Marculescu, and T.M. Stulnig. 2013. "Treatment with n-3 polyunsaturated fatty acids overcomes the inverse association of vitamin D deficiency with inflammation in severely obese patients: a randomized controlled trial," *PLoS One* 8(1):e54634.

Iyengar, B. 1998. "The hair follicle: a specialized UV receptor in the human skin?" *Biological Signals and Receptors* 7(3):188–94.

Jabbour, G., H.D. Iancu, and A. Paulin. 2015. "Effects of high-intensity training on anaerobic and aerobic contributions in total energy release during repeated supramaximal exercise in obese adults," *Sports Medicine–Open* 1(1):36.

Jastreboff, A.M., R. Sinha, C. Lacadie, D.M. Small, R.S. Sherwin, and M.N. Potenza. 2013 "Neural correlates of stress- and food cue-induced food craving in obesity: association with insulin levels," *Diabetes Care* 369(2):394–402.

Jimenez-Cruz, A. M. Bacardi-Gascon, W.H. Turnbull, P. Rosales-Garay, and I. Severino-Lugo. 2003. "A flexible, low-glycemic index Mexican-style diet in overweight and obese subject with type 2 diabetes improves metabolic parameters during a 6-week treatment period," *Diabetes Care* 26(7):1967–70.

Kadooka, Y., M. Sato, K. Imaizumi, A. Ogawa, K. Ikuyama, Y. Akai, M. Okano, M. Kagoshima, and T. Tsuchida. 2010. "Regulation of abdominal adiposity by probiotics (Lactobacillus gasseri SBT2055) in adults with obese tendencies in a randomized controlled trial," *European Journal of Clinical Nutrition* 64(6):636–43.

Kamezaki, F., S. Sonoda, Y. Tomotsune, H. Yunaka, and Y. Otsuji. 2010. "Seasonal variation in metabolic syndrome prevalence," *Hypertension Research* 33(6):568–72.

Kamran, A., S. Hanif, and G. Murtaza. 2015. "Risk factors of childhood asthma in children attending Lyari General Hospital," *Journal of the Pakistan Medical Association* 65(6):647–50.

Kasai, M., N. Nosaka, H. Maki, S. Negishi, T. Aoyama, M. Nakamura, Y. Suzuki, H. Tsuji, H. Uto, M. Okazaki, and K. Kondo. 2003. "Effect of dietary medium- and long chain triacylglycerols (MLCT) on accumulation of body fat in healthy humans," *Asia Pacific Journal of Clinical Nutrition* 12(2):151–60.

Kim, M.J., V. Pellioux, E. Guyot, J. Tordiman, L.C. Bui, A. Chevallier, C. Forest, C. Benelli, K. Clément, and R. Barouki. 2012. "Inflammatory pathway genes belong to major targets of persistent organic pollutants in adipose cells," *Environmental Health Perspectives* 120(4):508–14.

Knowlton, W.M., and D.D. McKemy. 2011. "TRPM8: From cold to cancer, peppermint to pain," *Current Pharmaceutical Biotechnology* 12(1):68–77.

Kong, L.C., J. Tap, J. Aron-Wisnewsky, V. Pelloux, A. Basdevant, J.L. Bouillot, J.D. Zucker, J. Doré, and K. Clément. 2013. "Gut microbiota after gastric bypass in human obesity: increased richness and associations of bacterial genera with adipose tissue genes," *American Journal of Clinical Nutrition* 98(1):16–24.

Koopman, F.A., S.P. Stoof, R.H. Straub, M.A. Van Maanen, M.J. Vervoordeldonk, and P.P. Tak. 2011. "Restoring the balance of the autonomic nervous system as an innovative approach to the treatment of rheumatoid arthritis," *Molecular Medicine* 17(9–10):937–48.

Korpela, K., H.J. Flint, A.M. Johnstone, J. Lappi, K. Poutanen, E. Dewulf, N. Delzenne, W.M. de Vos, and A. Salonen. 2014. "Gut microbiota signatures predict host and microbiota responses to dietary interventions in obese individuals," *PLoS One* 9(6):e90702.

Kräuchi, K., S. Reich, and A. Wirz-Justice. 1997. "Eating style in seasonal affective disorder: who will gain weight in winter?" *Comprehensive Psychiatry* 38(2):80–7.

Krueger, H., D. Turner, J. Krueger, and A.E. Ready. 2014. "The economic benefits of risk factor in Canada: tobacco smoking, excess weight, and physical inactivity," *Canadian Journal of Public Health* 105(1):e69–78.

Kummerow, F.A. 2009. "The negative effects of hydrogenated trans fats and what to do about them," *Atherosclerosis* 205(2):458-65.

Lachin, T. 2014. "Effect of antioxidant extract from cherries on diabetes," *Recent Patents on Endocrine Metabolic & Immune Drug Discovery* 8(1):67–74.

Landsberg, L. 2012. "Core temperature: a forgotten variable in energy expenditure and obesity?" *Obesity Reviews* 13 Supplement 2:97–104.

Lemmer, J.T., F.M. Ivey, A.S. Ryan, G.F. Martel, D.E. Hurlbut, J.E. Metter, J.L. Fozard, J.L. Fleg, and B.F. Hurley. 2001. "Effect of strength training on resting metabolic rate and physical activity: age and gender comparisons," *Medicine & Science in Sports & Exercise* 33(4):532–41.

Levy, A., A. Salamon, M. Tucci, C.L. Limebeer, L.A. Parker, and F. Leri. 2013. "Co-sensitivity to the incentive properties of palatable food and cocaine in rats; implications for co-morbid addictions," *Addiction Biology* 18(5):763–73.

Lewis M., P. Ghassemi, and J. Hibbeln. 2013. "Therapeutic use of omega-3 fatty acids in severe head trauma," *The American Journal of Emergency Medicine* 31(1):273.

Li, S., J.H. Zhao, J. Luan, R.N. Luben, S.A. Rodwell, K.T. Khaw, K.K. Ong, N.J. Wareham, and R.J. Loos. 2010. "Cumulative effects and predictive value of common obesity-susceptibility variants identified by genome-wide association studies," *American Journal of Clinical Nutrition* 91(1):184–90.

Li, D.K., M. Miao, Z. Zhou, C. Wu, H. Shi, X. Liu, S. Wang, and W. Yuan. 2013. "Urine bispenol-A level in relation to obesity and overweight in school-age children," *PLoS One* 18(6):e65399.

Lim, S., I. Sakuma, M.J. Quon, and K.K. Koh. 2014. "Differential metabolic actions of specific statins: clinical and therapeutic considerations," *Antioxidants and Redox Signaling* 20(8):1286–99.

Lin, X., G. Dong, Q. Wang, and X. Du. 2015. "Abnormal gray matter and white matter volume in 'internet gaming addicts,'" *Addictive Behavior* 40:137–43.

Liou, A.P., M. Paziuk, J.M. Luevano Jr., S. Machineni, P.J. Turnbaugh, and L.M. Kaplan. 2013. "Conserved shifts in the gut microbiota due to gastric bypass reduce host weight and adiposity," *Science Translational Medicine* 5(178):178ra41.

Lips, P., N.M. van Schoor, and R.T. de Jongh. 2014. "Diet, sun, and lifestyle as determinants of vitamin D status," *Annals of the New York Academy of Sciences* 1317:92–8.

Lloyd, L., and B. Miller. 2013. "The impact of seasonality on changes in body weight and physical activity in Mexican-American women," *Women and Health* 53(3):262–81.

MacKelvie, K.J., J.E. Taunton, H.A. McKay, and K.M. Khan. 2000. "Bone mineral density and serum testosterone in chronically trained, high mileage 40–55 year old male runners," *British Journal of Sports Medicine* 34(4):273–8.

Mailloux, R.J., M. Florian, Q. Chen, J. Yan, I. Petrov, M.C. Coughlan, M. Laziyan, D. Caldwell, D. Lalande, D. Patry, C. Gagnon, K. Sarafin, J. Truong, H. M. Chann, N. Ratnayake, N. Li, W.G. Willmore, and X. Jin. 2014. "Exposure to a northern contaminant mixture (NCM) alters hepatic energy and lipid metabolism exacerbating hepatic steatosis in obese JCR rats," *PLoS One* 9(9):e106832.

Manickam, B., T. Washington, N.E. Villagrana, A. Benjamin, S. Kukreia, and E. Barengolts. 2012. "Determinants of circulating 25-hydroxyvitamin D and bone mineral density in young physicians," *Endocrine Practice* 18(2):219–26.

Marachev, A., L. Solovenchuk, and A. Lapinski. 1992. "Adaptive changes of membrane lipid composition in humans living in the north," *Arctic Medical Research* 51(2):98–102.

Marin, M.F., J.K. Morin-Major, T.E. Schramek, A. Beaupré, A. Perna, R.P. Juster, and S.J. Lupien. 2012. "There is no news like bad news: women are more remembering and stress reactive after reading real negative news than men," *PLoS One* 7(10):e47189.

Martelli, D., M. Luppi, M. Cerri, D. Tupone, E. Perez, G. Zamboni, R. Amici R. 2012. "Waking and sleeping following water deprivation in the rat," *PLos One* 7(9):e46116.

Martins, C., M.D. Robertson, and L.M. Morgan. 2008. "Effects of exercise and restrained eating behavior on appetite control," *Proceedings of the Nutrition Society* 67(1):28–41.

Mathai, M.L., S. Naik, A.J. Sinclair, H.S. Weisinger, and R.S. Weisinger. 2008. "Selective reduction in body fat mass and plasma leptin induced by angiotensin-converting enzyme inhibition in rats," *International Journal of Obesity* (London) 32(10)1576–84.

Matossian-Motley, D.L., D.A. Drake, J.S. Samimi, C.A. Camargo Jr., and S.A. Quraishi. 2016. "Association between serum 25(OH)D level and nonspecific musculoskeletal pain in acute rehabilitation unit patients," *Journal of Parenteral and Enteral Nutrition* 40(3):367–73.

McAfee, A.J., E.M. McSorley, G.J. Cuskelly, A.M. Fearon, B.W. Moss, J.A. Beattie, J.M. Wallace, M.P. Bonham, and J.J. Strain. 2011. "Red meat from animals offered a grass diet increases plasma and platelet n-3 PUFA in healthy consumers," *British Journal of Nutrition* 105(1):80–9.

McCue, M.D. 2004. "General effects of temperature on animal biology," chapter from N. Valenzula and V.A. Vance, *Temperature Dependent Sex Determination* (Washington, DC: Smithsonian Books), 71–78.

McFadden, E., M.E. Jones, M.J. Schoemaker, A. Ashworth, and A.J. Swerdlow. 2014. "The relation between obesity and exposure to light at night: cross-sectional analyses of over 100,000 women in the Breakthrough Generations Study," *American Journal of Epidemiology* 180(3):245–50.

Meck, W.H., and R.M. Church. 1987. "Nutrients that modify the speed of internal clock and memory storage processes," *Behavioral Neuroscience* 101(4):465–75.

Melnik, B.C. 2015. "Milk: an epigenetic amplifier of FTO-mediated transcription? Implications for Western diseases," *Journal of Translational Medicine* 13:385.

Miller, G.D., B.J. Nicklas, C.C. Davis, C. Legault, and S.P. Messier. 2012. "Basal growth hormone concentration increased following a weight loss focused dietary intervention in older overweight and obese women," *Journal of Nutrition, Health, and Aging* 16(2):169–74.

Million, M., E. Angelakis, M. Paul, F. Armougom, L. Leibovici, and D. Raoult. 2012. "Comparative meta-analysis of the effect of Lactobacillus species on weight gain in humans and animals," *Microbial Pathogenesis* 53(2):100–8.

Mitchell, T.W., K. Ekrros, S.J. Blanksby, A.J. Hulber, and P.L. Else. 2007. "Differences in membrane acyl phospholipid composition between an endothermic mammal and an ectothermic reptile are not limited to any phospholipid class," *Journal of Experimental Biology* 210(pt 19): 3440–50.

Mohr, M., L. Nybo, J. Grantham, and S. Racinais. 2012. "Physiological responses and physical performance during football in the heat," *PLoS One* 7(6):e39202.

Molinaro, F., E. Paschetta, M. Cassader, R. Gambino, and G. Musso. 2012. "Probiotics, prebiotics, energy balance, and obesity: mechanistic insights and therapeutic implications," *Gastroenterology Clinics of North America* 41(4):843–54.

Mozaffarian, D., T. Hao, E.B. Rimm, W.C. Willett, and F.B. Hu. 2011. "Changes in diet and lifestyle and long-term weight gain in women and men," *New England Journal of Medicine* 364(25):2392–404.

Murosaki, S., T.R. Lee, K. Muroyama, E.S. Shin, S.Y. Cho, Y. Yamamoto, and S.J. Lee. 2007. "A combination of caffeine, arginine, soy isoflavones, and L-carnitine enhances both lipolysis and fatty acid oxidation in 3T3-L1 and HepG2 cells in vitro and in KK mice in vivo," *Journal of Nutrition* 137(10):2252–7.

Murphy, M., R. Samms, A. Warner, M. Bolborea, P. Barrett, M.J. Fowler, J.M. Brameld, K. Tsintzas, A. Kharitonenkov, A.C. Adams, T. Coskun, and F.J. Ebling. 2013. "Increased responses to the actions of fibroblast growth factor 21 on energy balance and body weight in a seasonal model of adiposity," *Journal of Neuroendocrinology* 25(2):180–9.

Neutelings, T., C. A. Lambert, B.V. Nusgens, and A.C. Colige. 2013. "Effects of mild cold shock (25°C) followed by warming up at 37°C on the cellular stress response," *PLoS One* 8(7):e69687.

Nishi, Y., H. Hiejima, H. Hosoda, H. Kaiya, K. Mori, Y. Fukue, T. Yanase, H. Nawata, K. Kangawa, and M. Kojima. 2005. "Ingested medium-chain fatty acids are directly utilized for the acyl modification of gherlin," *Endocrinology* 146(5)2255–64.

Ogur, R., H. Istanbulluoglu, A. Korkmaz, A. Barla, O.F. Tekbas, and E. Oztas. 2014. "Report: investigation of anti-cancer effects of cherry in vitro," *Pakistan Journal of Pharmaceutical Sciences* 27(3):587–92.

Oliver, G., and J. Wardle. 1999. "Perceived effects of stress on food choice," *Physiological Behavoir* 66(3):511–5.

Oppenheimer, G.M., and I.D. Benrubi. 2014. "McGovern's Senate Select Committee on Nutrition and Human Needs versus the meat industry on the diet-heart question (1976-1977)," *American Journal of Public Health* 104(1):59-69.

O'Rahilly, S., and I.S. Farooqi. 2006 "Genetics of obesity," *Philosophical Transactions of the Royal Society B: Biological Sciences.* 361(1471):1095-1105.

Orton, H.D., N.J. Szabo, M. Clare-Salzler, and J.M. Norris. 2008. "Comparison between omega-3 and omega-6 polyunsaturated fatty acid intakes as assessed by a food frequency questionnaire and erythrocyte membrane fatty acid composition in young children," *European Journal of Clinical Nutrition* 62(6):733–8.

Oshakbayev, K.P., K. Alibek, I.O. Ponomarev, N.N. Uderbayev, and B.A. Dukenbayeva. 2014. "Weight change therapy as a potential treatment for end-stage ovarian carcinoma," *American Journal of Case Reports* 15:203–11.

Pan, A., Q. Sun, J.E. Manson, W.C. Willett, and F.B. Hu. 2013. "Walnut consumption is associated with lower risk of type 2 diabetes in women," *Journal of Nutrition* 143(4):512–8.

Panter-Brick, C. 1995. "Inter-individual and seasonal weight variation in rural Nepali women," *Journal of Biosocial Science* 27(2):215–33.

Pare, P.W., and J.H. Tumlinson. 1999. "Plant volatiles as a defense against insect herbivores," *Plant Physiology* 121(2):325–32.

Park, K.S. 2010. "Raspberry ketone increases both lipolysis and fatty acid oxidation in 3T3-L1 adipocytes," *Planta Medica* 76(15):1654–8.

Plotnikoff, G.A., and J.M. Quigley. 2003. "Prevalence of severe hypovitaminosis D in patients with persistent, nonspecific musculoskeletal pain," *Mayo Clinic Proceedings* 78(12):1463–70.

Prentice, A.M., A.E. Black, W.A. Coward, and T.J. Cole. 1996. "Energy expenditure in overweight and obese adults in affluent societies: an analysis of 319 doubly-labeled water measurements," *European Journal of Clinical Nutrition* 50(2):93–7.

Quigley, E.M. 2013. "Gut bacteria in health and disease," *Gastroenterology and Hepatology* 9(9):560–9.

Ramírez-Vick, M., L. Hernández-Dávila, N. Rodríguez-Rivera, M. López-Valentín, L. Haddock, R. Rodríguez-Martínez, and A. González-Bossolo. 2015. "Prevalence of vitamin D insufficiency and deficiency among young physicians at University District

Hospital in San Juan, Puerto Rico," *Puerto Rico Health Science Journal* 34(2):83–8.

Reed, H.L. 1995 "Circannual changes in thyroid hormone physiology: the role of cold environmental temperatures," *Arctic Medical Research* 54 Supplement 2:9–15.

Reinehr, T. 2011. "Thyroid function in the nutritionally obese child and adolescent," *Current Opinion in Pediatrics* 23(4):415–20.

Reinehr, T., and W. Andler. 2002. "Thyroid hormones before and after weight loss in obesity," *Archives of Disease in Childhood* 87(4):320–3.

Rezapour, S., S. Najari, and N. Ghaemian. 2015. "The impacts of long-term intensive agriculture on the Vertisol properties in a calcareous region," *Environmental Monitoring and Assessment* 187(5):247.

Riebl, S.K., and B.M. Davy. 2013. "The hydration equation: update on water balance and cognitive performance," *ACSM's Health and Fitness Journal* 17(6):21-8.

Roecklein, K.A., J.A. Schumacher, M.A. Miller, and N.C. Emecoff. 2012. "Cognitive and behavioral predictors of light therapy use." *PLoS One* 7(6):e39275.

Romeijn N., R.J. Raymann, E. Møst, B. Te Lindert, W.P. Van Der Meijden, R. Fronczek, G. Gomez-Herrero, and E.J. Van Someren. 2012. "Sleep, vigilance, and thermosensitivity," *Pflügers Archiv - European Journal of Physiology* 463(1):169–76.

Ross, A. C. 2011. *Dietary Reference Intakes for Calcium and Vitamin D* (Washington, DC: National Academy Press).

Rozenberg S., J.J. Body, O. Bruyère, P. Bergmann, M.L. Brandi, C. Cooper, J.P. Devogelaer, E. Gielen, S. Goemaere, J.M. Kaufman, R. Rizzoli, and J.Y. Reginster. 2016. "Effects of dairy products consumption on health: benefits and beliefs--a commentary from the Belgian Bone Club and the European Society for Clinical and Economic Aspects of Osteoporosis, Osteoarthritis and Musculoskeletal Diseases," *Calcified Tissue International* 98(1):1-17

Rule, D.C., K.S. Broughton, S.M. Shellito, and G. Maiorano. 2002. "Comparison of muscle fatty acid profiles and cholesterol concentrations of bison, beef cattle, elk, and chicken," *Journal of Animal Science* 80(5):1202–11.

Sabbağ, C. 2012. "Seasonal BMI changes of rural women living in Anatolia," *International Journal of Environmental Research and Public Health* 9(4):1159–70.

Sade, M.Y., I. Kloog, I.F. Liberty, I. Katra, L. Novack, and V. Novack. 2015. "Air pollution and serum glucose levels: a population-based study," *Medicine* (Baltimore) 94(27):e1093.

Sahay, B., Y. Ge, N. Colliou, M. Zadeh, C. Weiner, A. Mila, J.L. Owen, and M. Mohamadzadeh. 2015. "Advancing the use of Lactobacillus acidophilus surface layer protein A for the treatment of intestinal disorders in humans," *Gut Microbes* 6(6):397–7.

Sanchez, M., C. Darimont, V. Drapeau, S. Emady-Azar, M. Lepage, E. Rezzonico, C. Ngom-Bru, B. Berger, L. Philippe, C. Ammon-Zuffrey, P. Leone, G. Chevrier, E. St-Amand, A. Marette, J. Doré, and A. Tremblay. 2014. "Effect of Lactobacillus rhamnosus CGMCC1.3724 supplementation on weight loss maintenance in obese men and women," *British Journal of Nutrition* 111(8):1507–19.

Saunders, A.G., J.P. Dugas, R. Tucker, M.I. Lambert, and T.D. Noakes. 2005. "The effects of different air velocities on heat storage and body temperature in humans cycling in a hot, humid environment," *Acta physiologica Scandinavica* 183(3):241–55.

Savcheniuk, O.A., O.V. Virchenko, T.M. Falalyeyeva, T.V. Beregova, L.P. Babenko, L.M. Lazarenko, O.M. Demchenko, R.V. Bubnov, and M.Y. Spivak. 2014. "The efficacy of probiotics for monosodium glutamate-induced obesity: dietology concerns and opportunities for prevention," *EPMA Journal* 5(1):2.

Schinzari, F., M. Tesauro, V. Rovella, N. Di Daniele, N. Mores, A. Veneziana, and C. Cardillo. 2013. "Leptin stimulates both endothelin-1 and nitric oxide activity in lean subjects but not in patients with obesity-related metabolic syndrome," *Journal of Clinical Endocrinology & Metabolism* 98(3):1235–41.

Schulman, C.I., N. Namias, J. Doherty, R.J. Manning, P. Li, A. Elhaddad, D. Lasko, J. Amortegui, C.J. Dy, L. Dlugasch, G. Baracco, and S.M. Cohn. 2005. "The effect of antipyretic therapy upon outcomes in critically ill patients: a randomized, prospective study," *Surgical Infections* (Larchmont) 6(4):369–75.

Schwieterman, M.L., T.A. Colquhoun, E.A. Jaworski, L.M. Bartoshuk, J.L. Gilbert, D.M. Tieman, A.Z. Odabasi, H.R. Moskowitz, K.M. Folta, H.J. Klee, C.A. Sims, V.M. Whitaker, and D.G. Clark. 2014. "Strawberry flavor: diverse chemical compositions, a seasonal influence, and effects on sensory perception," *PLoS One* 9(2):e88446.

Seifert, S.M., J.L. Schaechter, E.R. Hershorin, and S.E. Lipshultz. 2011. "Health effects of energy drinks on children, adolescents, and young adults," *Pediatrics* 127(3):511–28.

Serpa Neto, A., V.G. Pereira, G. Colombo, F.C. Scarin, C.M. Pessoa, and L.L. Rocha. 2014. "Should we treat fever in critically ill patients? A summary of the current evidence from three randomized controlled trials," *Einstein* (São Paulo) 12(4):518–23.

Sgoutas, D., and F.A. Kummerow. 1970. "Incorporation of trans-fatty acids into tissue lipids," *American Journal of Clinical Nutrition* 23(8):1111–9.

Shah, R.V., and A.B. Goldfine. 2012. "Statins and risk of new-onset diabetes mellitus," *Circulation* 126(18):e282–4.

Sharma A., M. Bemis, and A.R. Desilets. 2014. "Role of medium chain triglycerides (Axona®) in the treatment of mild to moderate Alzheimer's disease," *American Journal of Alzheimer's Disease and Other Dementias* 29(5):409-14.

Shook, R.P., G.A. Hand, C. Drenowatz, J.R. Hebert, A.E. Paluch, J.E. Blundell, J.O. Hill, P.T. Katzmarzyk, T.S. Church, and S.N. Blair. 2015. "Low levels of physical activity are associated with dysregulation of energy intake and fat mass gain over 1 year," *American Journal of Clinical Nutrition* 102(6):1332–8.

Shorten, A.L., K.E. Wallman, and K.J. Guelfi. 2009. "Acute effect of environmental temperature during exercise on subsequent energy intake in active men," *American Journal of Nutrition* 90(5):1215–21.

Siddiqui, A., S.V. Madhu, S.B. Sharma, and N.G. Desai. 2015. "Endocrine stress responses and risk of type 2 diabetes mellitus," *Stress* 18(5):498–506.

Simondon, K.B., T. Ndiaye, M. Dia, A. Yam, M. Ndiaye, A. Marra, A. Diallo, and F. Simondon. 2008. "Seasonal variations and trends in weight and arm circumference of non-pregnant rural Senegalese women, 1990–1997," *European Journal of Clinical Nutrition* 62(8):997–1004.

Sinha, R., and A.M. Jastreboff. 2013. "Stress as a common risk factor for obesity and addiction," *Biological Psychiatry* 73(9): 827–35.

Song, Z., L. Liu, A. Sheikhahmadi, H. Jiao, and H. Lin. 2012. "Effect of heat exposure on gene expression of feed intake regulatory peptides in laying hens," *Journal of Biomedicine and Biotechnology* 2012(4-5):484869.

St-Onge, M.P., and A. Bosarge. 2008. "Weight-loss that includes consumption of medium-chain triacylglycerol oil leads to a greater rate of weight and fat mass loss than does olive oil," *American Journal of Clinical Nutrition* 87(3):621–6.

Stubbs, R.J., N. Mazian, and S. Whybrow. 2001. "Carbohydrates, appetite, and feeding behavior in humans," *Journal of Nutrition* 131(10):2775S–2781S.

Su-Que L, M. Ya-Ning, L. Xing-Pu, Z. Ye-Lun, S. Guang-Yao, and M Hui-Juan. 2013. "Effect of consumption of micronutrient enriched wheat steamed bread on postprandial plasma glucose in healthy and type 2 diabetic subjects," *Nutrition Journal* 12:64

Sun, T., R.J. Long, Z.Y. Liu, W.R. Ding, and Y. Zhang. 2012. "Aspects of lipid oxidation of meat from free-range broilers consuming a diet containing grasshoppers on alpine steppe of the Tibetan Plateau," *Poultry Science* 91(1):224–31.

Sun, W.M., L.A. Houghton, N.W. Read, D.G. Grundy, and A.G. Johnson. 1988. "Effect of meal temperature on gastric emptying of liquids in man," *Gut* 29(3):302–5.

Sun, T., R.J. Long, Z.Y. Liu, W.R. Ding, and Y. Zhang. 2012. "Aspects of lipid oxidation of meat from free-range broilers consuming a diet containing grasshoppers on alpine steppe of the Tibetan Plateau," *Poultry Science* 91(1):224–31.

Susiarjo, M., I. Sasson, C. Mesaros, and M.S. Bartolomei. 2013. "Bisphenol-A exposure disrupts genomic imprinting in the mouse," *PLoS Genetics* 9(4):e1003401.

Tabata, I., K. Nishimura, M. Kouzaki, Y. Hirai, F. Ogita, M. Miyachi, and K. Yamamoto. 1996. "Effects of moderate-intensity endurance and high-intensity intermittent training on anaerobic capacity and VO2max," *Medicine & Science in Sports & Exercise* 28(10):1327–30.

Thorne, H.C., K.H. Jones, S.P. Peters, S.N. Archer, and D.J. Dijk. 2009. "Daily and seasonal variation in the spectral composition of light exposure in humans," *Chronobiology International* 26(5):854–66.

Torjusen, H., A.L. Brantsaeter, M. Haugen, J. Alexander, L.S. Bakketeig, G. Lieblein, H. Stigum, T. Naes, J. Swarts, G. Holmnoe-Ottesen, G. Roos, and H.M. Meltzer. 2014. "Reduced risk of pre-eclampsia with organic vegetable consumption: results from the prospective Norwegian mother and child cohort study," *BMJ Open* 4(9):e006143.

Trogdon, J. G., E.A. Finklestein, C.W. Feagan, and J.W. Cohen. 2012. "State- and payer-specific estimates of annual medical expenditures attributable to obesity," *Obesity* (Silver Spring) 20(1):214–20.

Turnbaugh, P.J., R.E. Ley, M.A. Mahowald, V. Magrini, E.R. Mardis, and J.I. Gordon. 2006. "An obesity-associated gut microbiome with increased capacity for energy harvest," *Nature* 444(7122):1027–31.

Urban, L.E., M.A. McCrory, H. Rasmussen, A.S. Greenberg, P.J. Fuss, E. Saltzman, and S.B. Roberts. 2014. "Independent, additive effects of five dietary variables on ad libitum energy intake in a residential study," *Obesity* (Silver Spring) 22(9):2018–25.

Uribarri, J., S. Woodruff, S. Goodman, W. Cai, X. Chen, R. Pyzik, A. Yong, G.E. Striker, and H. Vlassara. 2010. "Advanced glycation end products in foods and a practical guide to their reduction in diet," *Journal of the American Dietetics Association* 110(6):911–16.

van der Lans, A.A., J. Hoeks, B. Brans, G.H. Vijgen, M.G. Visser, M.J. Vosselman, J. Hansen, J.A. Jörgensen, J. Wu, F.M. Mottaghy, P. Schrauwen, and W.D. van Marken Lichtenbelt. 2013. "Cold acclimation recruits human brown fat and increase nonshivering thermogenesis," *Journal of Clinical Investigation* 123(8):3395–403.

Van Dycke, K.C., W. Rodenburg, C.T. van Oostrom, L.W. van Kerkhof, J.L. Pennings, T. Roenneberg, H. van Steeg, and G.T. van der Horst. 2015. "Chronically alternating light cycles increase breast cancer risk in mice," *Current Biology* 25(14):1932-7.

Van Elswyk, M.E., and S.H. McNeill. 2014. "Impact of grass/forage feeding versus grain finishing on beef nutrients and sensory quality: the U.S. experience," *Meat Science* 96(1):535–40.

Van Proeyen, K., K. Szlufcik, H. Nielens, M. Ramaekers, and P. Hespel. 2011. "Beneficial metabolic adaptations due to endurance exercise training in the fasted state," *Journal of Applied Physiology* (1985) 110(1):236–45.

Verma, D., J. Wood, G. Lach, H. Herzog, G. Sperk, and R. Tasan. 2016. "Hunger promotes fear extinction by activation of amygdala microcircuit," *Neuropsychopharmacology* 41(2):431–9.

Verreijen, A.M., S. Verlaan, M.F. Engberink, S. Swinkels, J. de Vogel-van den Bosch, and P.J. Weijs. 2015. "A high whey protein-, leucine-, and vitamin D-enriched supplement preserves muscle mass during intentional weight loss in obese older adults: a double-blind randomized controlled trial," *American Journal of Clinical Nutrition* 101(2):279–86.

Vimaleswaran, K.S., et al. 2013. "Causal relationship between obesity and vitamin D status: bi-directional Mendelian randomization analysis of multiple cohorts," *PLoS Medicine* 10(2):e1001383.

Voss, J.D., R.L. Atkinson, and N.V. Dhurandhar. 2015. "Role of adenoviruses in obesity," *Reviews in Medical Virology* 25(6):379–87.

Vrecer, M., S. Turk, J. Drinovec, and A. Mrhar. 2003. "Use of statins in primary and secondary prevention of coronary heart disease and ischemic stroke. Meta-analysis of randomized trials," *International Journal of Clinical Pharmacology and Therapeutics* 41(12):567–77.

Wegmann, M., O. Faude, W. Poppendieck, A. Hecksteden, M. Fröhlich, and T. Meyer. 2012. "Pre-cooling and sports performance: a meta-analytic review," *Sports Medicine* 42(7):545–64.

Westerterp, K.R., and J.R. Speakman. 2008. "Physical activity energy expenditure has not declined since the 1980s and matches energy expenditures of wild mammals," *International Journal of Obesity* (London) 32(8):1256–63.

Wideman, L., J. Weltman, M.L. Hartman, J.D. Veldhuis, and A. Weltman. 2002. "Growth hormone release during acute and chronic aerobic and resistance exercise: recent findings," *Sports Medicine* 32(15):987–1004.

Wilding, J.P. 2002. "Neuropeptides and appetite control," *Diabetic Medicine* 19(8):619–27.

Wrangham, R.W., J.H. Jones, G. Laden, D. Pilbeam, and N. Conklin-Brittain. 1999. "The raw and the stolen. Cooking and the ecology of human origins," *Current Anthropology* 40(5):567-94.

Wu, J., S. Dong, G. Liu, B. Zhang, and M. Zheng. 2011. "Cooking process: a new source of unintentionally produced dioxins?" *Journal of Agricultural and Food Chemistry* 59(10):5444-9.

Wu, T., C. Yao, L. Huang, Y. Mao, W. Zhang, J. Jiang, and Z. Fu. 2015. "Nutrients and circadian rhythms in mammals," *Journal of Nutritional Science and Vitaminology* (Tokyo) 61 Supplement:S89-91.

Young, L.R., and M. Nestle. 2002. "The contribution of expanding portion sizes to the U.S. obesity epidemic," *American Journal of Public Health* 92(2):246-9.

Young, L.R., and M. Nestle. 2007. "Portion sizes and obesity: responses of fast-food companies," *American Journal of Public Health* 28(2):238-48.

Zhang, Q., Y. Su, and J. Zhang. 2013. "Seasonal difference in antioxidant capacity and active compounds contents of Eucommia ulmoides oliver leaf," *Molecules* 18(2):1857-68.

Zhang, Y., T. Neogi, C. Chen, C. Chaisson, D.J. Hunter, and H.K. Choi. 2012. "Cherry consumption and decreased risk of recurrent gout attacks," *Arthritis & Rheumatology* 64(12):4004-11.

Zofková, I., and R.L. Kancheva. 1995. "The relationship between magnesium and calciotropic hormones," *Magnesium Research* 8(1):77-84.

Glossary

Adipose tissue: fat tissue

Adrenaline: a stress hormone that is secreted by the adrenal gland that increases heart rate, pulse rate, and blood pressure, and raises the blood levels of glucose and lipids.

Adipocyte: fat cell

Advanced glycation end-product (AGE): proteins or lipids that become glycated (have sugars attached to them chemically) as a result of exposure to excess sugars or high temperature cooking. They can be a factor in aging and in the development or worsening of many degenerative diseases, such as diabetes, atherosclerosis, chronic renal failure, and Alzheimer's disease.

Aerobic: requiring oxygen, or relating to exercise that is intended to improve the efficiency of the body's cardiovascular system in absorbing and transporting oxygen

Alpha melanocyte-stimulating hormone (alpha-MSH): pituitary hormone that helps in the development of pigment in skin but also reduces appetite and increases satiety/ fullness with eating

Anaerobic: Not requiring oxygen, or relating to exercise that creates an oxygen debt such as weight lifting

Antimicrobial: substance that kills bacteria

Antioxidant: a substance such as a vitamin that inhibits oxidation (the binding of oxygen to chemicals in food and the body) which can have harmful or damaging effects

Apoptosis: programmed cell death designed as a way to prevent abnormal cells such as cancer from growing

Attention deficit hyperactivity disorder (ADHD): any of a range of behavioral disorders occurring primarily in children, including such symptoms as poor concentration, hyperactivity, and impulsivity

Betaine: a sweet-tasting alkaloid that occurs in the sugar beet and other plants and in animals that helps in detoxifying certain substances and functions as a methyl donor in methylation

Bisphenol A (BPA): a synthetic organic compound used in the manufacture of epoxy resins and other polymers such as plastic used in plastic water bottles which can have activity in the body like a synthetic form of the hormone estrogen.

Body mass index (BMI): a weight-to-height ratio, calculated by dividing one's weight in kilograms by the square of one's height in meters and used as an indicator of obesity and underweight. $Kg/m2$

Brown adipose tissue (BAT): Brown fat's main function is to generate body heat. Human newborns and hibernating mammals have high levels of brown fat. Recently found to play a role in adult weight loss as well.

Calcitonin gene-related peptide (CGRP): this is a nerve derived signaling chemical, which is elevated in obesity and dilates blood vessels. It is thought to play a potential role in development of migraines and other conditions associated with obesity.

Cardiovascular: The system of the heart and blood vessels.

Cholecystokinin: is a peptide hormone of the gastrointestinal system responsible for stimulating the digestion of fat and protein by causing the gallbladder to squeeze and empty bile into the intestines.

Choline: is an essential nutrient derived from such things as egg yolks and is important in the making and movement of fats in the body. It is particularly important in formation of cell membranes. It is also important in memory and muscle control.

Circadian: running on a twenty-four-hour cycle, even in the absence of light fluctuations.

Cortisol: is a steroid hormone, meaning that it is made from cholesterol. It is produced in the adrenal gland and released in response to stress and low blood-glucose. It increases blood sugar, suppresses the immune system, and aids the metabolism of fat, protein, and carbohydrates.

Demethylation: Removal of a methyl chemical group from a section of DNA. Some areas of the DNA are inactivated when this happens, meaning they don't get copied and turned into the final protein machinery the DNA codes for. Other areas of the DNA can be activated by demethylation.

Deoxyribonucleic acid (DNA): The copyable material present in all animals and plants as the main constituent of genetic information in the chromosomes. Provides the blueprint for available characteristics for that organism.

Dioxin: a highly toxic compound produced as a byproduct in some manufacturing processes, notably herbicide production and paper bleaching. Also results from high temperature cooking of certain foods. Thought to be a contributor to both cancer and obesity risk.

Diverticulitis: inflammation of a diverticulum (small hernia-like outpouching of the colon wall caused by poor diet), causing pain and disturbance of bowel function.

Dopamine: a compound present in the body as a neurotransmitter that gives the rewarding sensation of pleasure during certain activities or when certain foods are eaten, it is also a precursor of other substances including epinephrine.

Endorphin: Hormones that activate the body's opiate receptors, causing an analgesic or pain-reducing as well as a pleasure effect. Frequently cited as released with exercise.

Enzyme: substance (usually protein) produced by a living organism that acts as a catalyst to increase a specific chemical reaction in the body, such as breaking down certain nutrients during digestion.

Epinephrine: a hormone released by the adrenal medulla in response to stress, anger, or fear. It is the "fight or flight" hormone and acts to increase heart rate, blood pressure, cardiac output, and carbohydrate metabolism. In other words, it causes blood sugar to rise as a rapidly available fuel source within the blood stream by increasing production in the liver, increasing release from muscle glycogen, and reducing insulin sensitivity.

Genetically modified organism (GMO): an organism whose genetic material has been altered artificially so that its DNA contains genes not normally found in that organism. Certain crops, such as corn and soybeans, are frequently genetically modified. This is different from normal selection of crops done in the past where existing characteristics were naturally preferred by plant, flower, or fruit selection and cross-pollination by a farmer.

Ghrelin: an enzyme produced by stomach lining cells that stimulates appetite. It is one of the main hunger hormones.

Glucagon: a hormone produced in the pancreas that breaks down glycogen to glucose in the liver. Released when blood sugars are low. Considered the opposite hormone to insulin.

Glycated hemoglobin: Hemoglobin with sugar chemically attached. It is referred to as HbA1c and is measured primarily to identify the three-month average blood glucose concentration since the lifespan of red blood cells where hemoglobin is found is three months.

Glycation: This is the bonding of a protein or fat molecule with a sugar molecule, such as fructose or glucose. This can be worse when blood sugar levels are higher. This can change the shape and function of the fat or protein molecule increasing risk for disease and more rapid signs of aging. Glycation may occur either inside the body (endogenous glycation) or outside the body (exogenous glycation) during cooking processes.

Glycemic index: This is a system that ranks foods on a scale from 1 to 100 based on their effect on blood-sugar levels compared to eating pure glucose. The higher the index number the more of an impact it has on insulin secretion and potential weight gain.

Gluconeogenesis: New sugar formation occurring in the liver in response to hormones, exercise or stress.

High-density lipoprotein (HDL): "Good cholesterol". Lipoproteins are combinations of fats (lipids) and proteins, which is the form in which lipids are transported in the blood. HDLs transport cholesterol from the tissues of the body to the liver, so the cholesterol can be eliminated in the bile.

High intensity interval training (HIIT): exercise strategy alternating short periods of very intense anaerobic exercise with less-intense recovery periods

Hippocampus: portion of the brain, thought to be the center of emotion, memory, and the autonomic nervous system

Homeostasis: the body's tendency to maintain a condition of balance or equilibrium within its internal environment, even when faced with external changes

Hyperglycemia: excess blood sugar usually in diabetics

Hypothalamus: portion of the brain that coordinates both the autonomic nervous system and the activity of the pituitary and controls body temperature, thirst, hunger, sleep and emotional activity.

Hypothyroid: condition where the thyroid hormone levels are too low to maintain normal metabolism

Leptin: a protein produced by fatty tissue and believed to regulate fat storage in the body

Light-at-night (LAN): artificial light exposure after sunset

Low-density lipoprotein (LDL): "bad cholesterol". The form of lipoprotein that transports cholesterol in the blood.

Macronutrient: food substance required in large amounts by animals that include carbohydrates, protein and fat.

Medium chain triglyceride (MCT): These are fats consisting of between six and twelve carbon chains. The four most common are: Caproic Acid, Caprylic Acid, Capric Acid, and Lauric Acid. All are found in coconut oil with Lauric Acid being the most healthy and prominent component. They are also found in human milk, and the first three acids occur in goat's milk (capra = goat).

Melatonin: a hormone in vertebrate animals that is derived from serotonin. It is secreted by the pineal gland especially in response to darkness, and has been linked to the regulation of wake-sleep cycles. Retinal exposure to light decreases secretion.

Mellitus: honey sweetened. Usually used in the term "Diabetes mellitus" to refer to the condition where blood sugar levels are elevated beyond normal leading to many medical complications.

Methylation: DNA methylation is a process by which methyl groups are added to DNA. Methylation modifies the function of the DNA. If methylation occurs in a gene promoter (the part of the DNA at the beginning of a gene), it usually turns off the gene. This is thought to be one of the ways that nature selects dad or mom's genes to be active.

Microbiome: the microorganisms (bacteria, viruses, fungi and parasites) in a particular environment including the body

Micronutrient: food substance such as a vitamin, mineral, or phytonutrient that is found in minute quantities but is necessary for normal growth, development, health, or survival.

MicroRNAs (miRNAs): These are a class of small noncoding RNA (meaning they don't get translated to form proteins) that bind to mRNAs (messenger RNA) resulting in posttranscriptional regulation of gene expression. In other words, miRNAs can make a gene be more expressed.

Mitochondria: an organelle found in most cells, in which the biochemical processes of respiration and energy production happens. Cells that have higher energy use such as heart muscle and liver have more mitochondria.

Monosodium glutamate (MSG): a compound that occurs naturally as a breakdown product of proteins and is used as a flavor enhancer in food which makes food taste richer, meatier and heartier. It has become a very common food additive and is called by many names including: yeast extract, hydrolyzed yeast extract, autolyzed yeast, glutamate, textured protein, yeast nutrient, calcium caseinate, glutamic acid, yeast food, hydrolyzed protein. Many products contain it.

Neuropeptide substance P: Neurotransmitter substance that has been associated with the regulation of inflammation, satiety, vasodilation, mood disorders, anxiety, stress, reinforcement, neurogenesis, respiratory rhythm, neurotoxicity, pain, and nociception. Can be increased by sunlight exposure. Is a current research target as a possible weight loss agent.

Neurotoxin: Any substance that is toxic or damaging to nerve cells or brain tissue.

Neurotransmitter: A chemical substance released at the end of a nerve fiber in response to a nerve impulse that causes the transfer of the impulse to another nerve fiber, a muscle fiber, or other structure.

Obesogen: Any chemical substance in the environment that can promote fat gain and obesity by altering lipid homeostasis and fat storage, changing metabolic setpoints, disrupting energy balance or modifying the regulation of appetite and satiety.

Parasympathetic nervous system (PNS): The part of the involuntary nervous system that serves to slow the heart rate, increase intestinal and glandular activity, and relax the sphincter muscles. Serves to run the normal functions of digestion and reproduction and is usually in opposite function to the "fight-or-flight" hormones of the sympathetic system.

Peptide YY: substance released by the last segment of the small intestine and the colon in response to feeding that decreases appetite. Y is the single letter abbreviation for the amino acid tyrosine, so it is also referred to as "peptide tyrosine tyrosine". Often low in obesity.

Phosphatidylcholine: Also called lecithin. Is a component of cell membranes and thought to play a role in cell signaling and repair.

Phytochemical: chemicals naturally produced by plants that may serve a role in growth, defense or repair within the plant.

Phytonutrient: substances found in plants believed to provide a benefit to human health and help prevent various diseases.

Post-traumatic stress disorder (PTSD): A condition of persistent mental and emotional stress as a result of injury or severe psychological shock, typically involving disturbance of sleep and constant vivid recall of the experience, with dulled responses to others and to the outside world.

Prebiotic: A non-digestible food ingredient that promotes the growth of beneficial microorganisms in the intestines.

Probiotic: Bacteria introduced into the body for their health benefits.

Rapid eye movement (REM): The rapid jerky eye movements during dream stages of the sleep cycle.

Seasonal affective disorder (SAD): depression associated with late autumn and winter and thought to be caused by a lack of light. Can be treated by bright light exposure. Characterized by depressed mood, lethargy, increased appetite, weight gain and cravings for carbohydrates.

Serotonin: neurotransmitter that is partially responsible for feelings of happiness, contentment and social acceptance. Can suppress appetite in the brain and alter how fat is burned in the rest of the body.

Serum triglyceride: measured blood fat levels.

Sleep apnea: disorder in which a person has pauses in breathing or shallow breathing while sleeping. Usually associated with obesity and snoring.

Steatohepatitis: fat accumulation in liver associated with inflammation of the liver.

Suprachiasmatic nuclei (SCN): part of the hypothalamus of the brain, above the optic chiasma (where the optic nerves of the eyes join) that regulates the circadian rhythm.

Sympathetic nervous system (SNS): part of the autonomic nervous system that decreases secretions, increases heart rate, increases blood pressure and causes pupillary dilation. "Fight-or-flight" system dependent on epinephrine.

T-cell: a white blood cell involved in immunity produced or processed by the thymus gland.

Testosterone: a steroid hormone (made from cholesterol) that stimulates development of male secondary sexual characteristics such as pubic and axillary hair, body shape, sexual organ growth, odor and deep voice, produced mainly in the testicles, but also in the ovaries and adrenal cortex.

Thermogenic: producing heat through metabolic stimulation.

Triglyceride: main constituents of natural fats and oils. When elevated in the blood can be a sign of increased risk for stroke and heart disease.

Interesting Facts

1. Drinking water will increase your resting energy expenditure enough to result in greater than 2.2 pounds (one kilogram) per year of weight loss.
2. Cold stimulates appetite up to twenty percent.
3. Cold slows metabolism by as much as 15% by eliminating more thyroid hormone.
4. Heat is a natural appetite suppressant.
5. Exercise in heat burns thirty percent more calories than exercise in cold.
6. Lack of light and vitamin D can cause increased calorie intake by twenty-six percent and slow metabolism (less calorie use) by thirteen percent.
7. Modern light has decreased the average hours of sleep from nine down to seven.
8. Periodontal disease, along with obesity, increases risk of cardiovascular disease by as much as fifteen percent.
9. Adequate vitamin D levels can drop the risk of obesity by eleven percent.
10. Food additives such as emulsifiers can cause irritable bowel and weight gain.
11. Light-at-night (LAN) causes weight gain and contributes to risk of cancer and depression.

Resources

Fast-Track Your Health: The Four Keys to Successful Weight Loss by Mohammad A. Emran, MD

For your personal health improvement plan and for further advice on planning and ensuring success in a weight loss effort. This book gives you practical advice on the four elements that people who succeed with weight loss and keep the weight off permanently have in common. Use these techniques along with this book to not only silence your fat gene but guarantee success in achieving any weight loss goal.

http://www.grassrootshealth.net/media/download/
For glycemic indices of food.

http://localfoods.about.com/od/finduselocalfoods/a/ natlseason.htm
To find locally grown, in-season foods and their harvest seasons.

http://www.usana.com
You may have noticed that I mentioned "high quality supplements" in the book and you may be wondering what to use. The reality is that this question can be a daunting one if you don't know where to look or what products to rely on. After over three years of research and three years of personal experience with amazing results for my family and patients, I feel confident in the quality and outcomes with USANA brand products since they are guaranteed to have 100% of what is on the label and are scientifically based. For a health assessment that can tell you which USANA supplements might be

right for you go to **USANA True Health Assessment.** Don't try to get them anywhere other than the official USANA links or websites since distributors are not authorized to sell them on other online markets. That means products on anything other than the official sites can be expired or counterfeit!

https://www.livestrong.com
For great, easy to read health information, news, blogs, and tips. While some of their stories are on somewhat trendy topics, they can give you a good starting place to learn on a topic. By no means in depth, comprehensive, or definitive on any subject but good for getting a superficial understanding quickly.

http://eatingacademy.com
To get into the deep science descriptions of how metabolism works, how your body uses energy, and potential ways to take advantage of this during exercise.

https://seanknows.wordpress.com
If financial or personal challenges are interfering with your success.

https://www.vitamindcouncil.org
For the benefits of vitamin D and the risks of not having enough.

http://www.sucrose.com/lref.html
For more about sugar.

http://www.SpringCure.com
SpringCure is my company where we practically apply all the book materials in online and in live coaching workshops. For a bunch of free resources go to **springcure.com/resources** where you will find:
1. When fruits and vegetables are in season and what their health benefits are
2. To get your free Goal Setting Guide to help you set what you want to achieve.
3. A printable "Fat Gene Trigger" Guide
4. For health and weight loss coaching go to www.SpringCure.com

5. To set up a live workshop for a group or to create a weight loss challenge at work see the "Contact Us" section on Spring-Cure.com

6. Like SpringCure on Facebook and Twitter to get up-to-date videos, blogs and inspiration or to ask your questions.